D1034571

SEX AND NUTRITION

SEX AND NUTRITION

A modern study of nutritional aspects
of sexuality

by PAAVO O. AIROLA, N.D.

Published by
INFORMATION, INCORPORATED
NEW YORK, NEW YORK

PRINTED IN THE UNITED STATES OF AMERICA

TABLE OF CONTENTS

INTRODUCTION
by Frank S. Caprio, M.D.

FOREWORD:

PART ONE: GLANDS HOLD THE SECRET OF SEXUAL POWER

Chapter 1: *The relationship between nutrition and sex "rediscovered" by modern science*
"Old wives' tales" in a new scientific light • New biological approach • How nutrition affects your sex life • Aphrodisiacs and modern science

Chapter 2: *Glands—the mysterious hormone laboratories*
Glands control and regulate all life-processes • Two kinds of glands, exocrine and endocrine

Chapter 3: *How glands control your sex life*
The pituitary gland • The thyroid gland • The adrenals • The parathyroids • The pancreas and the Islands of Langerhans • Thymus • Magic internal laboratories

Chapter 4: *Female reproductive system and its functions*
The female sex organs • Vulva • Clitoris • Hymen • Accessory glands • Vagina • Breasts • The Uterus • Ovaries—the female sex glands • Female sex hormones • How Mrs. L. regained her youth

Chapter 5: *Male reproductive system and its functions*
The male sex organs • Penis • What causes impotence • Prostate gland • Other male sex organs • The testes • Male sex hormones • Nutrition and sexual virility

PART TWO: SEX AND NUTRITION

Chapter 6: *Is nutrition the whole answer?*
Various causes of sexual disorders: inhibitions, ignorance, social taboos, fears, boredom, etc.

Chapter 7: *"Since the beginning of time . . ."*
Aphrodisiacs—what they are • True and false aphrodisiacs • Asia—the center of the art and the science of love • China and Japan • Arabian countries • Europe and Middle East • Premature ejaculation and the "Staying Power" • Ancient aphrodisiacs in the light of modern science

Chapter 8: *High-protein diet and sex*
"High-protein craze" and how it originated • What are proteins • How much protein do we actually need • Fads and fallacies about proteins • Do you need meat for sexual virility? • Libido-destroying additives in meat • How to plan a high-virility diet with a minimum of animal proteins

Chapter 9: *How vitalizing nutrition can build a basis for healthy and happy sex life*
Fads and facts about nutrition • Why universal disagreement on the question: what is man's proper diet • What is I.S.R.N.V.S. • Natural foods spell optimum health and freedom from disease • Living foods for peak of health and vitality • Enzymes—the miracle life-force • Enzymes and virility • Poisons in food can harm your health and lower your virility • Poisons and sexual health • Five basic rules of nutrition for optimum health and a healthy and happy sex life • Instant or long-term virility

Chapter 10: *How vitamins, minerals, and trace elements affect your sex life*
Vitamins and minerals for sexual power • How prevalent are vitamin deficiencies • How to fortify your diet with vitamins • Minerals and trace elements • How to get a maximum of vitamins, minerals, and trace elements in your diet

Chapter 11: *Ten special foods that may maintain and enhance your sexual vigor*
"Special" foods for sexual vigor • Not aphrodisiacs

but excellent sources of potent nutrition • 1. Wheat germ • 2. Wheat germ oil • 3. Sesame seeds • 4. Honey • 5. Raw nuts and seeds • 6. Milk • 7. Kelp • 8. Fish liver oil • 9. Lecithin • 10. Eggs

PART THREE: SEX AFTER FORTY

Chapter 12: *How to prevent premature aging.*
Life-long potency is man's birthright • Other factors affecting man's virility after 40 • Does obesity diminish sexual libido • Male and female menopause may be favorably affected by proper nutrition • How to prevent sexual senility with improved nutrition

Chapter 13: *Can prostate problems be prevented by nutritional means?*
What causes prostate disorders? • Can prostate disorders be prevented? • Zinc and prostate disorders • Seven-point program for prevention of prostate disorders.

Chapter 14: *How sex affects your heart*
Heart disease and sex • "Death on top of tummy" • Should individual with heart disease engage in sexual activity? • Heart, sex, and nutrition • Your heart and vitamin E • Your heart and vitamin C • Other nutritional factors • Nutritional program for stronger heart

Chapter 15: *"If he kissed you once . . ."*
Often seemingly insignificant things can interfere with full enjoyment of sex • Halitosis almost nonexistent • What causes bad breath • How odorous and toxic wastes are eliminated • Constipation—the common cause of bad breath • Morning breath • How to prevent and eliminate bad breath—without mouthwash

PART FOUR: SEX IN A CHEMICALIZED WORLD

Chapter 16: *Are synthetic hormones in food turning American men into eunuchs?*
How Italian playboys lost their masculinity • What is stilbestrol and how does it cause sexual disorders • Other chemicals in meat

Chapter 17: *Can smoking cause impotence?*
Researchers agree—excessive smokers can become impotent

Chapter 18: *What about alcohol and sex?*
Alcohol and potency • Alcohol—health destroyer • Beer and wine • Alcoholism and sex • Nutrition, alcohol, and sex

Chapter 19: *Can insecticides cause sterility in people?*
How insecticides affect fertility • DDT and sex hormones

Chapter 20: *What causes malformed babies?*
Fast growing American problem • "Acts of God" or results of modern chemicalized way of life? • Nutritional deficiencies and congenital anomalies

Chapter 21: *How safe is "The Pill"?*
The Pill and thrombo-embolic disease • The Pill and liver damage • The Pill and frigidity • Other adverse side-effects

Chapter 22: *Can air pollution cause reproductive disorders and decline in fertility?*
Effects of lead poisoning • Was the fall of Rome caused by lead poisoning? • How serious is lead poisoning in the United States? • Russia prohibits lead in gasolines • How can you protect yourself from lead poisoning

CONCLUSION: A new basis for physical, emotional and sexual health.

INTRODUCTION

by Frank S. Caprio, M.D.

The author, Paavo Airola, N.D., famed European nutritionist, is to be congratulated for his efforts to show how nutrition influences sexuality. He writes with authority, having acquainted himself with the latest scientific knowledge in his special field. His premise is that man is what he eats and what he eats is capable of influencing his virility; hence the average man is able to add years to his sex life through the use of natural and enriched foods. This premise is based on the fact that certain foods high in vitamin and mineral content have virility-enhancing qualities.

Potency, in many instances, may be weakened by nutritional deficiencies. Virility is also dependent on numerous other factors such as exercise, physical health, adequate amount of sleep, mental attitude and ability to relax. Physical and mental health go hand in hand to produce the individual who can function in a normal manner.

An outsize waistline acquired from overeating and physical indolence is bound to play a major role in impotence problems during later years. But I have encountered a number of patients between seventy-five and eighty years old who reported that they were able to function adequately.

Nevertheless, there is a need today for further scientific research into the relationship of certain special foods to sexual vitality. It is also gratifying to know that the author gives hope to the many men and women who wish to revitalize their sexual activity and achieve sexual longevity.

I feel the book merits wide distribution.

Frank S. Caprio, M.D.
Washington, D.C.
September 5, 1969

FOREWORD

As the title suggests, this study is limited to the nutritional aspects of sexuality. It will furnish a practical guide in the modern use of nutritional knowledge to prevent sexual disorders and correct malfunctions. You can improve your sex life through diet—but only if you have the requisite information.

Books on various aspects of sex are available in growing numbers. Human sexuality has become a legitimate subject for scientific inquiry. Dr. Alfred C. Kinsey, of the Institute For Sex Research at Indiana University, established that fact for our times. The last decade has witnessed a rapidly increasing amount of research in this vital aspect of man's total personality.

In St. Louis, Missouri, The Reproductive Biology Research Foundation, under the direction of Dr. William B. Masters, is committed to study the physiological and biological aspects of sex.

Many other groups are working in various American and European research centers toward the same end.

The breakthrough in sex education has resulted in many books on the subject. Most of these deal with the psychological and emotional aspects of sex. Indisputably, psychological and emotional factors are the underlying causes of many sexual disorders. But conviction is growing among specialists in the field that many seemingly emotional problems have nutritional origins. As for the more obviously physiological disorders—impotency, frigidity, male or female sterility, miscarriage, menstrual pain and menopausal distress—the evidence is fairly clear.

The purpose of this work is not to stimulate a healthy individual into greater sexual activity through improved nutrition or any other means. Rather, we want to help those who are not enjoying their full potential in their physical expression of love.

Modern science sees sexuality as part of the total personality. Properly understood and directed it ought to be used as "responsibly and creatively as any other human faculty," according to Dr. Mary Steichen Calderone, of the Sex Information and Education Council of the United States. We do not subscribe to the idea that increased sex education and open discussion will help the cause of so-called "new morality." Sex instinct and desire are God-given gifts. Sexual expression is one of the deepest forms of human communication. Ignorance in sex matters has caused needless unhappiness and frustration to millions. Frankness in discussion is imperative in understanding problems and finding the remedial solutions.

I do not pretend that improved nutrition in itself will guarantee sexual contentment. Many other factors are involved. But the relationship between nutrition and sexuality is a definitely established scientific fact.

In this book I will show you:

- How mysterious little chemical laboratories within your body—your endocrine and sex glands—control your sexual life and are directly responsible for the healthy function or malfunction of your sex organs.
- How you may be able to stimulate these glands for youthful vitality, increased virility and sex appeal.
- How vital, scientific nutrition can bring you not only better general health, but also a healthier sex life.
- How you can use ten special foods and natural and harmless food substances, which are scientifically and/or empirically proven capable of stimulating your sex glands and improving your sexual vigor.
- How prostate problems after middle age may be avoided by nutritional means.

- How female and male menopause can be postponed and a satisfying sex life enjoyed after fifty—sixty—or one hundred years of age.

In the following chapters you will find answers to such questions as:

- How does alcohol affect your sexuality?
- Can smoking cause impotence in men?
- Can air pollution cause decline in fertility?
- How does sexual activity affect your heart?
- Can insecticides cause sterility?
- Are synthetic hormones in meat causing impotence in men?

The answers to these questions and many more may surprise and even shock you. If only one of the dozens of suggestions in this book can help you to achieve a more satisfying sex life, then you will be richly rewarded for the effort of reading it.

The scientific quest into this fascinating field of nutrition and sex has just started. The last word has not been said. However, enough has been discovered to enable you to benefit from intelligent application. As Plato, the ancient thinker, said, "Virility of the body and mind are one. Whoever destroys the virility of the body harms the soul, too." Improving your sex life will have a profound effect on your whole personality. You may achieve, through greater peace of mind, new success in your profession or career. In whatever fashion, an improved sex life will bring you greater happiness.

CHAPTER 1

THE RELATIONSHIP BETWEEN SEX AND NUTRITION "RE-DISCOVERED" BY MODERN SCIENCE

ONLY TEN YEARS ago this book could not have been written—for two reasons. *First,* our western civilization was still under the thwarting influence of Victorian taboos on sex. Although our double-standard society has long been wallowing in eroticism and has been widely exploiting sex in literature, movies, and television, it was unwilling to recognize sex as a legitimate subject for open scientific discussion. And *second,* in spite of a widespread popular conviction that there is a relationship between nutrition and sex, modern medical science derided such ideas as nonsense and superstition.

Now our western culture is experiencing a sexual revolution. Attitudes are changing. The chains of taboos and inhibitions are being broken. As yet no one seems sure that this change is for the better. But one thing is sure—man's sexuality has become a legitimate subject for scientific research and inquiry. As researchers delve into the physiological aspects of sex, nutrition is coming into the limelight as a vitally important factor. Doctors have stopped laughing at the relationship between food and sex and have begun serious investigation.

"OLD WIVES' TALES" IN A NEW SCIENTIFIC LIGHT

Many so-called "old wives' tales" about food and sex, once ridiculed by anyone with a claim to education, can now be substantiated with the newest scientific research. Doctors have learned that some folk remedies, which have survived for thousands of years, should not be discarded lightly. Our most effective modern drugs—penicillin, aspirin, digitalis, atropine and quinine, to name a few—are contemporary forms of folk remedies that were used before germs were discovered.

A few short decades ago, medical thinking was centered in pasteurian philosophy. According to that philosophy, the cause of disease is invasion by hostile bacteria. With that reference frame, health is no more than freedom from invasion. Even now, it is not uncommon for a doctor to ignore the relationship between a patient's nutrition and his ailment. An examination by a physician of this school will involve no inquiry into nutritional habits. What the patient eats, or does not eat, are left out of the record.

Fortunately, this kind of doctor is disappearing. An informed modern doctor is aware that health is related to environmental factors, including nutrition. The pendulum has in fact swung the other way for some, who boldly declare that most health disorders and diseases can be traced to poor eating habits.

NEW BIOLOGICAL APPROACH

The advance of biological medicine has had a stimulating effect on progressive research. Doctors are beginning to realize that most of man's ills are the result of prolonged abuse of elementary health rules. The role of nutrition in preventive and therapeutic medicine has become increasingly evident. Biochemical imbalance in the tissues, derangement in the metabolic processes due to faulty dietary patterns, are recognized as major causative factors in many chronic and degenerative diseases.

Nutritional imbalances and deficiences may affect every aspect of man's physical and mental well-being. The normal function of every organ and gland is dependent on adequate and proper nutrition. Man's sexual system and its functions are no exception to this rule. Doctors have become increasingly aware that the quality of nutrition determines the state of sexual health. Men's and women's sexual desires and abilities, and the healthy function of their reproductive systems, are to a significant degree dependent on the nutritional quality of the foods they eat.

HOW NUTRITION AFFECTS YOUR SEX LIFE

Just why and how does nutrition play so important a role in your sex life? How does it affect your sexual capacity, your virility and your fertility?

Your sexual life is directed by your glandular system. The glands directly responsible for sexual activity are the so-called endocrines. Most of your body's functions are controlled by them. The hormones produced by the endocrine and sex glands hold the secret of your sexual power.

The female sex hormone, *estrogen,* plays a vital part in the life pattern of every woman. Not only the health of her reproductive system, the normal menstruations and pregnancies, but her general physical well-being and her mental and psychic attitudes, are affected by this sex hormone.

Testosterone, the male sex hormone, plays an equally important part in man's sexual life and his general health. These hormones and other secretions of the endocrine glands are the *spark plugs* that provide stimulus and drive for the body as well as the mind. The healthy function of the endocrine glands and sufficient production of hormones are indispensible to healthy functioning of the sex organs.

Dr. James H. Leathem, of the Bureau of Biological Research at Rutgers University, believes that connective factors link your nutrition, your general health, the functional integrity of your endocrine system and your sexual desires and capability. The quality of your nutrition influences the synthesis, the quantity and the release of the endocrine hormones, which, in turn, directly and indirectly influence your libido and your sexual capacity.

Unadulterated and unrefined food, from which vital nutritive elements have *not* been removed or destroyed by processing, is essential for the healthy function of your glands. Our present-day devitalized foods, from which vital nutritive factors have been removed, and which, in addition, are loaded with many toxic preservatives and chemical additives, are not only destroying our health generally but are turning our men into sexual weaklings. Our diet habits relate to the increased number of miscarriages and the birth of malformed babies in our nation. The effect of malnutrition on the reproductive system is more powerful than many of us imagine.

Sex glands need specific nutrients—minerals, vitamins, and natural chemicals—in order to function properly. For example, the trace mineral *zinc* has been found indispensible for the health of the prostate gland. Without sufficient zinc in your diet, your prostate will degenerate. Vitamin B_1, thiamine, stimulates your sex glands indirectly through its action on the pituitary gland. Vitamin E is of paramount importance for your sexual health. These special nutrients are found in wheat germ oil, pumpkin and sunflower seeds, milk and other foods which I will describe in detail in Chapter 11. The regular use of these foods will have a beneficial effect on your sexual vigor.

APHRODISIACS AND MODERN SCIENCE

The foods recommended in this book *are not aphrodisiacs*. They are harmless sources of necessary nutrients. Further, all nutritional factors advocated in this book for your sexual health will benefit your general health as well.

We do not believe in artificial, chemical, or drug stimulation of the sex glands and organs, internally or externally, into unnatural accelerated activity. We subscribe to the first principle of healing, enunciated by the Father of Medicine, Hippocrates, twenty-five hundred years ago: *Primum est nil nocere*—the most important consideration is that the *treatment must do no harm*. The glands in the human body are extremely delicate and sensitive. They could easily cause physical and emotional harm if subjected to artificial stimulation. Therefore, we do not advocate any kind of synthetic hormone treatments, or other drugs. *Everything recommended in this book is harmless—natural foods and food substances, used and time-tested by countless generations of men and women and/or proven to be effective in modern research by reputable nutritionists and doctors.*

The working premises are simple:

- Proper nutrition is singularly the most important environmental factor affecting your health.
- The health of your sexual and reproductive system is tied to and directly dependent on the general health of your body and, thus, on your nutrition.
- Endocrine glands—these mysterious chemical laboratories in your body—hold the secret of your sexual power, libido and proper functions of your reproductive organs. The hormones and other secretions produced by these glands are the spark plugs that trigger and stimulate not only your sexual activity, but dramatically affect your general well-being, both physically and mentally.
- To assure the proper functioning of these vital glands and a generous supply of the all-important hormones, you must feed your glands with all the nutrients they need for effective and trouble-free activity throughout life.

Thus, the power to determine your sexual health is in your hands. Proper nutrition is the modern tool—and, paradoxically, also the oldest tool—with which you may correct your sexual inadequacies, and revitalize your physical, emotional, and sexual health.

The application of modern nutritional knowledge, right in your own kitchen, may supply you with solutions to dwindling sexual potency, female coldness, "bedroom fatigue," premature abortions, decreased fertility and the fear of congenital abnormalities which haunts our western world.

BRIEF SUMMARY OF CHAPTER 1

1. The "sexual revolution" of the last few decades is changing the attitude of responsible scientists toward sex. Man's sexuality has suddenly become a legitimate subject for scientific research and inquiry.
2. Although most of the research done so far has approached sex from the psychological and sociological viewpoint, a growing number of researchers have been delving into physiological and biological aspects of sexuality.
3. The relationship between nutrition and sex, formerly ridiculed as "old wives' tales," is now recognized by many doctors in the medical profession as being based on scientific facts.
4. Your endocrine glands are the "spark plugs" of your sexual desires. The hormones produced by these glands hold the secret of your amatory prowess.
5. The activity of these glands may be stimulated by proper nutrition and special nutritive substances. These harmless food substances can help your glands to reach the peak of their activity, increase your sexual vigor and help you to achieve a fuller and more satisfying sex life.

CHAPTER 2

GLANDS—THE MYSTERIOUS HORMONE LABORATORIES

SMALL ORGANS WITHIN your body control your physical and mental health, your sexual drive and fertility, your ambitions and attitudes, your emotions and feelings. These tiny and tireless workers, on which your health and well-being so totally depend, are your glands.

Glands serve many functions. There are glands that lubricate the mucous membranes which line your mouth, nose and internal organs. Your sweat glands regulate the temperature of your body and help to remove poisons from the system. Sebaceous glands produce an oily substance called sebum, which is essential for the healthy growth of your hair. Glands in your stomach produce enzymes for the proper digestion of food. Even such familiar organs as kidneys and liver are actually large glands. Kidneys are your most vital detoxicative glands. They extract from the blood metabolic waste products and eliminate them via urine. The liver is perhaps the most versatile gland in your body. It secretes bile, which is stored in the gall bladder and is used to digest fats. It stores glucose and B vitamins, acts as a blood filter and is involved in the blood-building processes. The pancreas, another digestive gland, produces insulin which is responsible for proper sugar metabolism in your body. When the insulin-productive capacity of the pancreas is weakened, the result is diabetes.

Lymphatic glands keep microbes from entering your bloodstream. There are mammary glands that secrete milk; lacrimal glands that secrete tears; the prostate gland which secretes seminal fluid; testes that manufacture sperm. Small and large, the glands number in the hundreds of thousands. Some, like the sweat glands, are microscopically small; while the liver is the largest gland in your system.

TWO KINDS OF GLANDS

Roughly, your glands can be divided into two groups. One group pours its secretions through a system of ducts into various parts of the body to perform their vital functions. These are *exocrine* glands, producing external secretions. The other group, the *endocrine* glands, is without discharge tubes or ducts. The substances secreted by them are poured directly into the blood; they do not reach either external or internal surfaces of the body and are, therefore, glands of internal secretion.

The endocrine glands are the *pituitary, pineal, adrenals, thyroid, parathyroid, thymus, pancreas, ovaries* and *testes*. These glands secrete chemical substances known as *hormones*. Hormones are released directly into the blood and are carried with the bloodstream to different parts of your body to regulate, stimulate or trigger its functions.

Some glands do not fit into this simple generalized division. The pancreas, for example, is involved in both exocrine and endocrine activity.

GLANDS CONTROL AND REGULATE ALL LIFE PROCESSES

This short outline of your glandular system may suffice to impress upon you that your glands are indeed important. Not only do they regulate all your physiological processes and functions, but they also control, influence and determine your entire personality and mental make-up. Your glands determine whether you are emotionally stable or disoriented, energetic or lethargic, agreeable or choleric, cold or temperamental. Your glands may be responsible if you are irritable, critical, nagging, or if your disposition is cheerful, tolerant and forgiving.

It stands to reason that you should do all you can to assure the healthy function of these vital miracle-workers—your glands—which have such a profound effect on your life and your personality. Luckily, you don't have to leave the quality of their performance to chance. Modern researchers have found that the healthy function of your glands is dependent to a great degree on your nutrition. Your glands can function properly only if they are supplied with all the nutritive elements they need: vitamins, minerals, proteins, essential fatty acids, trace elements, enzymes and natural hormones. These nutritive substances can come only from the foods you eat. By selecting proper foods and balancing your diet you can feed your glands for greater vitality, assure that they will give you trouble-free service and keep you vigorous throughout your long life. In the following chapters you will learn how to achieve that kind of optimum nutrition.

BRIEF SUMMARY OF CHAPTER TWO

1. Glands—the tiny chemical laboratories within your body—control and direct all your life processes.
2. Your glands are responsible for your physical and mental health, your sexual drive and fertility, your feelings and attitudes.
3. There are two kinds of glands—exocrine and endocrine. Endocrine glands are involved directly with your sex life.
4. It is in your power to keep these miracle chemical laboratories in top working condition.

CHAPTER 3

HOW GLANDS CONTROL YOUR SEX LIFE

ASK YOURSELF these questions:

Do you enjoy vibrant health and sparkling vitality? Not just a few happy moments now and then, but all the time?

Do you enjoy complete sexual fulfillment and happiness in your marriage? Is your wife—or husband—happy too?

Are you warm and affectionate, responsive and easy to live with?

Do you have initiative and zest for work and play, sustained optimistic interest and outlook on life, plenty of instant energy and youthful enthusiasm for your work and your favorite interests?

Are you satisfied with the way you look: your figure, your hair, your complexion, your waistline?

If you can answer all the above questions in the affirmative, this book is not for you. You are apparently one of the fortunate who have all the blessings that others dream about.

But if your answer to most of the above questions is *no,* then you had better look into the condition of your glands

—they may be responsible for your not feeling at par most of the time; for your mesotrophy, or half-health; for your chronic bedroom fatigue; for your lost interest in work and play; for your lack of enthusiasm and zest for life; for your chronic state of general dissatisfaction, pessimism, disappointment and frustration. Your neglected, malnourished and atrophied glands may be responsible for your deteriorating physical and mental condition.

Your endocrine glandular system controls not only the way you feel, but also the way you look. Premature signs of aging, early appearance of a wrinkled complexion, disappearing lips, loss and graying of hair, double chin, bulging waistline, loose and flabby skin on arms and legs—all these can be signs of insufficiently functioning endocrine glands. Glands possess a magic power which affects your whole being. They can make you old or young, ugly or beautiful, energetic or lethargic, virile or impotent. Don't you think it would be worth your while to take care of these omnipotent laboratories which have such a profound effect on your life?

Later in the book we will discuss in detail how you can feed your glands for increased beneficial results, but first let us learn what they are and how they work.

THE PITUITARY GLAND

This minute gland, weighing only six-tenths of a gram and about the size of a pea, is located at the base of the brain. Notwithstanding its small size, the pituitary is often called the master gland of the endocrine system. It manufactures ten or more specialized hormones with more complex and vital functions than those of the other endocrine hormones. Pituitary hormones control the functioning of all other endocrine glands, including the sex glands. The thyroid, the adrenals and the insulin-producing pancreas will all degenerate if the pituitary is removed.

The pituitary regulates the growth of the tissues and the bones. The "pituitary dwarf," miniature man, and the "pituitary giant," man who develops more rapidly than others from early childhood, are both a result of the defective action of the pituitary.

The pituitary secretes hormones which regulate the metabolism of water and salts, blood pressure, muscle constriction in childbirth, and kidney function. The pituitary is involved in anabolism (the building up of protoplasm); and one of the hormones secreted by the intermediate pituitary lobe possibly helps to determine skin color. Another pituitary hormone induces and stimulates the production of milk during nursing. Pituitary hormones control the storage and distribution of fat; gross obesity may be a result of pituitary imbalance.

Inadequate function of the pituitary gland may make you extremely sensitive to colds and infections, depress your appetite, and lower your resistance to stress. In older people, a degenerating pituitary gland causes loss of energy and lack of initiative. The disordered function of the pituitary may cause such diverse symptoms as an abnormal craving for sweets and underdeveloped sex organs.

The pituitary gland is involved in protecting you during crises. At the onset of stress, the pituitary secretes hormones ACTH and STH and speeds them through the blood to other glands, the adrenals, which rapidly produce adrenal hormones to meet the emergency situation.[1]

The pituitary gland has both a direct and an indirect effect on the sexual and reproductive organs. The work of Dr. Ascheim-Zondek and other researchers shows that the pituitary produces a hormone which acts directly on sex organs and on the secondary sex characteristics. This

[1] Selye, H., THE STRESS OF LIFE, McGraw-Hill, New York, 1956

substance, called pituitary gonadotrophic hormone, influences the germinal glands, stimulating them into production. If the pituitary gland fails, sexual development will be retarded and sexual maturity never attained. The pituitary influences the sex glands in both men and women. The testes produce spermatozoa and male sex hormones, and the ovaries produce ova and female sex hormones under direct stimulus from the pituitary gland.

Pituitary deficiency is associated with underdevelopment of the genital organs or so-called fatty degeneration. An under-functioning pituitary can bring about premature sexual aging and premature menopause by adversely affecting the ovaries. In men, a defectively functioning pituitary may result in premature impotence.

Although the pituitary is not in itself considered a sex gland, its influence on the sexual organs and their functions is so profound that it deserves all the attention and care necessary to assure its healthy activity.

The health of the pituitary is largely dependent on adequate nutrition. Research by Drs. Ershoff, Hurley, Rosenkrantz and others has demonstrated that vitamin E and vitamin B-complex, particularly such B-vitamins as riboflavin (B_2), pantothenic acid and choline are required to assure normal pituitary hormone production.[2] Complete proteins are also necessary. It is interesting to note that vitamin E is more concentrated in the pituitary gland than in any other part of the body. Research has shown that pituitary hormones cannot be produced in sufficient amounts without an ample supply of vitamin E in the diet. The effect of vitamin E on the pituitary is direct: first, it supplies an essential nutrient involved in hormone production; second, it protects the pituitary and the adrenal hormones from destruction by oxygen.[3] Vitamin E is well-known anti-oxidant.

---

[2] Davis, Adelle, LET'S GET WELL, Harcourt, Brace and World, Inc., New York, 1965

[3] Verzár, F., *International Congress on Vitamin E,* 1955

Foods rich in nutrients needed for the healthy function of the all-important pituitary—the master gland of your body—are: milk and cheese, whole grain products, raw nuts and seeds, wheat germ, citrus fruits and green vegetables. These are rich in B-complex vitamins, including pantothenic acid, choline and riboflavin. Brewer's yeast is an excellent food supplement and so is liver —they contain all the B-vitamins and are excellent sources of complete proteins which are essential for the healthy function of your pituitary gland. Milk and cheese are excellent sources of all the essential amino acids, the building blocks of proteins. For vitamin E, wheat germ and wheat oil are the best natural sources. The other cold-pressed vegetable oils, such as corn oil, safflower oil and sunflower oil are also good sources of vitamin E. But they must be cold-pressed and unprocessed, unlike the regular supermarket type.

THE THYROID GLAND

The thyroid gland is located in the foreground of the throat. Its important role is to govern the pace of your physical and mental life. The thyroid produces hormones which stimulate the oxygen consumption of all the body tissues, regulate growth, and control the body's metabolism.

The thyroid gland is of specific importance in your sexual life. An underactive thyroid gland can contribute to diminished sexual capacity. On the other hand, an overactive thyroid can overstimulate your sex glands. A weak or lazy thyroid can turn a young active man into a seemingly old man who has lost his initiative and interest in sex. The insufficient secretion of the thyroid hormone, *thyroxin,* slows down metabolic rate and contributes to obesity. Thyroxin contains considerable amounts of iodine, the lack of which can cause goiter.

Weak thyroid production can cause chronic fatigue, mental sluggishness, difficulty in concentration, depression and apprehension. The health of your hair, nails and complexion are affected by the thyroid. An underactive thyroid may also cause excessive menstruation.

An overactive thyroid is considered toxic. Sometimes the gland becomes overactive in attempting to compensate for nutritional deficiencies. Large amounts of iodine, 4 to 6 mg. a day and up to 500 mg. of vitamin E have been given in cases of hyperthyroidism (overactive thyroid) with success.[4] It has been demonstrated that iodine deficiency can cause goiter and even cancer of the thyroid.

Nutritional deficiencies can also cause an underactive thyroid. Both vitamin B_1 deficiency and deficiency in iodine can lower the activity of the thyroid gland.

How can you tell if your thyroid gland functions normally? Thyroid deficiency symptoms are: decreased libido, irregular and/or profuse menstruation, chronic fatigue, inability to concentrate, headaches, mental sluggishness and unjustified fears and worries. If you suspect thyroid deficiency, begin to feed your thyroid gland properly. Make sure your diet is rich in B-vitamins, especially vitamin B_1. Foods rich in B-complex vitamins are wheat germ, brewer's yeast, liver, whole grain products, nuts, beans and dairy products. For iodine, use kelp (seaweed) or iodized salt, preferably seasalt. Vitamin E is also important. It has been shown that vitamin E taken together with iodine has greatly increased the iodine absorption and the production of hormones by an underactive thyroid gland.[4] Wheat germ oil is the richest natural source of Vitamin E.

THE ADRENALS

The adrenals are located just above each of your kidneys. They are shaped somewhat like Brazil nuts, and

[4] Costa, A., et al., *International Congress on Vitamin E,* 1955

each one consists of two portions—*cortex* and *medulla*. The adrenal glands produce several hormones with a variety of functions.

Adrenalin, a "hormone of survival," is produced by the medulla and poured into the bloodstream in time of danger, in anger, fear, or other emotional excitement. Adrenalin governs the vegetative nervous system. It accelerates heart action and increases blood pressure and the sugar content of the blood. Adrenalin can slow up or stop your digestion, dilate the pupils of your eyes and cause your hair to stand on end.

The adrenal cortex produces a set of entirely different hormones. *Cortisone* is the best known and, perhaps, the most essential for your life. Cortisone plays many known and some unknown roles in metabolism. It has a demonstrated effect on rheumatoid arthritis, allergic disorders, rheumatic fever and inflammatory diseases of the skin and eyes. Insufficiency of the adrenal cortex hormones causes Addison's disease.

Aldosterone, another adrenal cortex hormone, is vitally involved in mineral metabolism and utilization, especially of the minerals sodium (salt), potassium and chlorine. It also helps your body to utilize fats, sugars and proteins. Aldosterone is also related to the action of sex hormones and has a profound effect on your sexual activity.

Still another adrenal hormone is called *desoxycortisone,* or DOC. It balances the effect of cortisone and regulates its action. DOC also helps your body to fight infections.

It is also believed that a variety of steroid substances secreted by the adrenal cortex are involved in such diverse conditions as cancer, mental diseases, and graying of the hair.

Prolonged nutritional deficiencies and stresses can cause what is called adrenal exhaustion. According to the famed authority on stress, Canadian doctor Hans Selye of the University of Montreal, any condition that harms or damages the body, physically or emotionally, is defined as a stress. Nutritional deficiencies, overwork, infections, lack of rest or exercise, poisonous substances in food and environment, separately or collectively, can cause *adrenal exhaustion.*

Nutritional deficiencies in particular affect the adrenal cortex adversely. Pantothenic acid (one of the B-vitamins) deficiency can cause a definite decrease in the production of adrenal hormones; and prolonged, severe deficiency of pantothenic acid can cause a complete stoppage in the production of cortisone and other adrenal hormones. Deficiencies of vitamins A, B_2 and E were also found to have an adverse effect on hormone production and even to cause degeneration of the adrenal cortex. Deficiency of linoleic acid and other essential fatty acids resulted in decreased production of adrenal hormones in human volunteers subjected to experiments.

The effect of such nutritional deficiencies can be easily avoided or corrected by fortifying your diet with foods or food supplements which are abundant in them. In severe deficiencies, of course, vitamins in tablet form should be used. Vegetable oils, such as cold-pressed corn oil and safflower oil, are rich in linoleic acid and other essential fatty acids. Dessicated liver and brewer's yeast are the best sources of B-complex vitamins. Wheat germ oil is the best natural source of Vitamin E.

Vitamin C is an extraordinarily effective ally in the treatment of virtually any condition caused by disease or stress. Even an adrenal exhaustion condition is favorably affected by large doses. Clinical tests have demonstrated that 500 milligrams of Vitamin C a day greatly stimulated the adrenal glands and markedly increased the adrenal hormone production in elderly hospitalized patients.[5]

[5] Smolyanski, B. L., *Fed. Proceedings,* 22, T1173, 1963

THE PARATHYROIDS

Four tiny oval glands are located at the upper and lower ends of each lobe of the thyroid gland. They secrete a hormone known as *parathormone,* the main known function of which is the regulation of the calcium and phosphorus supply to the blood and tissues. These glands are the parathyroids.

Calcium is important to practically all organs, bones and tissues of your body. A decreased calcium level in the blood stream can cause painful cramps and spasms. An adequate calcium and phosphorus supply is needed for strong bones and teeth, as well as for healthy nerves. Calcium is known as a natural "quietner" of the nervous system.

Phosphorus is an equally vital mineral. It is called the colleague of calcium, because calcium cannot do its job of building good bones and teeth, or nourishing the nerves, without a properly balanced supply of phosphorus in the bloodstream. Phosphorous is brain nutrient. It nourishes the brain cells and is used in increased amounts by those who are engaged in strenuous mental work. Phosphorus is also involved in hair growth and in carbohydrate and fat metabolism. A phosphorus deficiency may cause retarded growth, general weakness and reduced sexual powers.[6] Sufficient vitamin D is imperative for the proper assimilation of these minerals from the foods you eat.

The best sources of calcium and phosphorus are milk and cheese, whole grains, beans, nuts and most vegetables and fruits. Cod liver oil is a good source of vitamin D.

---

[6] Kordel, Lelord, EAT YOUR TROUBLES AWAY, Belmont Books, N. Y.

THE PANCREAS AND THE ISLANDS OF LANGERHANS

The *pancreas* is located near the kidneys and is considered a digestive organ. It secretes pancreatic juice which contains hormones and enzymes for the digestion and assimilation of proteins, starches and fats.

The *Islands of Langerhans* are clusters of granular cells scattered in the pancreas, but having a completely different, specialized function. They are named after the German physician, Dr. Paul Langerhans, who identified them in 1921. Canadian investigators, Drs. Frederick G. Banting and Charles H. Best, isolated the active agent of the pancreatic islands, now known as *insulin,* which regulates the amount of sugar in the blood. Glucose, or blood sugar, is the energy food for all body cells. The release of too much or too little glucose to the blood may cause grave illness and complete chaos in the function of the whole organism.

When the Islands of Langerhans are damaged they do not produce adequate amounts of insulin. Glucose accumulates in the blood and is excreted with urine as waste. This is the condition called diabetes. The United States, according to estimates, has no less than two and a half million diabetics.

Although the exact causes of diabetes are not known, it is considered by many doctors that improper diet, malabsorption, and other physiological stresses are involved, as suggested by Dr. H. Curtis Wood, Jr., M.D.[7] It has been demonstrated that excessive consumption of sugar and other refined carbohydrates will overwork the pancreas and may be responsible for development of the disease.

Diabetes has frequently responded well to nutritional treatments. Research by such scientists as Drs. S.N. Gershoff, Y. Kotake, and others, have shown that diabetics are usually

[7] Wood, H. Curtis, Jr., M.D., OVERFED BUT UNDERNOURISHED, Exposition Press, New York, 1959

deficient in vitamin B_6 and magnesium. It is known that white sugar and refined carbohydrates (white flour) rob the body of B-vitamins. Also, it has been demonstrated that vitamins C, B_{12}, E and lecithin are involved in diabetes. Conversely, Swedish researcher, Dr. Hjorth, has found that vitamin C can markedly increase the output of insulin.[8]

THYMUS

Knowledge about the *thymus* is comparatively recent. This two-lobed gland is located just below the thyroid. The thymus, large at birth, degenerates when puberty sets in and practically disappears in adults. The thymus plays an essential role in early normal growth. It is also involved in defense against infections. The thymus manufactures special cells that help build immunity.

Once the thymus was considered a useless organ. However, research by American, British and Swedish scientists have linked thymus malfunction to such diseases as leukemia, pernicious anemia, rheumatoid arthritis and rheumatic heart disease. Some cancer researchers believe that even cancer may be the result of breakdown in the immunological system which is controlled by the thymus.[9]

MAGIC INTERNAL LABORATORIES

The description of the endocrine glands in this chapter is intended to show you that these glands control and influence you all your life, through the minute quantities of chemical substances which they secrete. Not only are your mental and physical activities controlled by

---

[8] Hjorth, P., *Acta Medicae Scandinaviae,* 105, 67, 1940

[9] Maisel, A. Q. THE "USELESS" GLAND THAT GUARDS OUR HEALTH, *Reader's Digest,* November, 1960

these laboratories, but they directly influence your sexual activity as well.

There are other glands in your body, which we have not discussed as yet, which have a direct effect on your sex life. These specialized glands are directly involved in sexual urge and reproduction. They are called the *gonads,* or the male and female *germinal glands.* We will discuss them and their functions in the next two chapters.

BRIEF SUMMARY OF CHAPTER THREE

1. The endocrine glands, with their magic effect on your mind, your health and your sex life, are the pituitary, adrenals, thyroid, parathyroid, thymus, pancreas and gonads.
2. Functions and malfunctions of endocrine glands.
3. Hormone deficiencies and how they affect you.
4. Nutritional means of improving glandular activity, increasing hormone production and preventing glandular malfunctions.

CHAPTER 4

FEMALE REPRODUCTIVE SYSTEM AND ITS FUNCTIONS

MOST ENDOCRINE GLANDS described in the preceeding chapter are *indirectly* related to your sexual life and performance. In addition to these, your body is equipped with specific glands which are *directly* involved with reproduction and sexual activity. These are the *testes* in men and the *ovaries* in women. They are called the *gonads* in both sexes, or the *germinal glands.*

These glands are important not only for the reproductive processes but also to your mental and physical health. Let us familiarize ourselves with the female reproductive system and its functions.

THE FEMALE SEX ORGANS

The female sexual system consists of the external genitals, *vulva* (*labia majora* and *labia minora*), *clitoris* and *hymen;* and the internal sex organs, *ovaries, Fallopian tubes* leading from the ovaries, the *uterus* or womb, and the *vagina. Bartholin's glands* and *Skene's glands* are considered accessory.

Female breasts, or *mammary glands,* are also a part of the reproductive systems.

The female sexual organs may be divided into two groups according to their function:

1. The reproductive or generative organs.
2. The organs of copulation.

The organs of copulation are the vulva and the vagina. The generative organs are ovaries, Fallopian tubes, uterus and mammary glands. The vagina is considered both copulative and reproductive organ. It is the channel of intercourse and also the birth canal through which new life enters the world.

VULVA

The external female genitals, or *vulva,* consist of large and small "lips", or *labia,* and the *clitoris.* The outer or large lips, *labia majora,* are elongated folds of fatty tissue covered with hair in the adult woman. The inner, or small lips, *labia minora,* are thinner folds of tissue, which are for the most part covered with mucous membrane. The inner lips cover the opening into the *vagina* at the lower end, and the orifice of *urethra* at the upper end. The *clitoris* is located where the small lips meet.

CLITORIS

The word *clitoris* means "key" and is of Greek origin. The clitoris, an erected tissue which resembles the glans of the penis, is usually a quarter inch long. It may enlarge to an inch when subjected to sexual stimulation. The most erogenous part of the female body, the clitoris is the key to a woman's sexuality.

The clitoris is abundantly supplied with sensitive nerve

endings that channel sexual excitement. When engorged with blood and increased in size this organ evinces a miniature "erection." The result is closer contact with the male organ during sexual intercourse.

HYMEN

The *hymen,* or maidenhead, a thin membrane that partly covers the opening of the vagina, usually bursts during the first sexual act. However, in some females the membrane may be so thick that operative intervention is required before intercourse is possible.

The shape of the hymen varies greatly. It may have only one opening for menstrual discharge, or it may be perforated like a sieve. When the hymen is torn during first intercourse, the classic bleeding results.

Hymen, it is believed, has a two-fold purpose—to prevent sexual intercourse before sexual maturity and to inhibit the male seminal fluid from flowing out of the vagina. Even after the hymen is deflorated (torn), its remnants on the edges of the vaginal opening may serve to retain semen and increase the chance of conception.

ACCESSORY SEX GLANDS

The glands which secrete mucus during sexual excitation are *Skene's glands,* located near the opening of the uretha into the vaginal vestibule, and *Bartholin's glands,* near the vaginal opening. In addition, the inner lining of the vagina secretes lubrication during the sexual act.

There is disagreement among authorities on the exact function of these accessory glands. In non-human female mammals, these glands attract the male by secreting odorous substances. Is the same true of the human female? It may well be that these glands have a multiple purpose.

For satisfactory sexual intercourse, these lubricating glands must function properly, producing what is known as sexual wetness. When these natural lubricants are missing, an artificial lubricant may be used to make the penis penetrate easier. After the initial penetration is accomplished, the vagina is lubricated partly by mucous secretion from the uterus and vaginal walls, partly from secretions of the penis.

VAGINA

The *vagina,* which serves as the organ of intercourse and also as the birth canal, is a tubular cavity from three to six inches long with the shape of a bottle, narrowed in diameter at the exterior entrance, and widened at the interior. At the posterior end, the vaginal vault leads into the mouth of the uterus. The walls of the vagina are made of muscle tissue that can stretch considerably during childbirth. The mucous membranes which cover these muscles have great elasticity. A series of folds, which make distention possible, increase friction during sexual intercourse and serve to intensify sensation.

BREASTS

The female breasts, or *mammary glands,* contain from fifteen to twenty tiny canals which all lead to the nipple. These ducts are connected to the lactic glands which produce milk. At the beginning of puberty, fatty tissues fill the space between the ducts and cause the breasts to rise and enlarge. Breasts should reach their full development during pregnancy.

Perhaps more than the other sex glands, the breasts are directly affected by the quality and the quantity of nutrition. A proper diet, rich in all essential nutritive elements, is essential for sufficient production of milk during nursing. By the way, the size of breasts is not necessarily indicative of their capacity for milk production. Often large breasts contain much fat and a small number of lactic glands; while smaller breasts may have little fat, but a large number of lactic glands.

THE UTERUS

The *uterus,* or womb, is the central organ of the female reproductive system. Here the fertilized ovum settles in the mucous membrane and new life starts. The womb has a pear-like shape and is located just above and slightly behind the bladder. The narrower end of the pear, the cervix or neck of the womb, opens into the vagina. At the upper end, two oviducts, or Fallopian tubes, open into the uterus. These tubes bring the egg cell from the ovaries, to implant itself in the uterine wall. The uterine wall is a powerful muscle, one of the strongest in the body, powerful enough to hold a full-grown infant and then to expel it when the time comes.

The uterus is a delicate and intricate organ with many functions. Its monthly cycle or ovulation and menstruation is greatly influenced by hormones of the sex and endocrine glands. The uterus can be the site of many female troubles.

It has been demonstrated that many female troubles can be prevented and corrected by nutritional therapies. Premenstrual tensions, irregular menstruations, excessive or scanty menstruation, vaginal discharge, menopausal difficulties—all these have often been found to originate in a malfunctioning glandular system caused by faulty nutrition. These conditions have been corrected by nutritional therapies and special additions of vitamins and minerals to the diet. (More on nutritional treatment of female disorders in the following chapters.)

OVARIES—THE FEMALE SEX GLANDS

The *ovaries* are the most important organs of the female reproductive system. These, the female gonads, release ova that perpetuate the human race. They consist of two small glands, each the size and shape of an almond, situated on both sides of the uterus. The ovaries perform two jobs—to prepare the ova, or human eggs, and thus make pregnancy possible; and to secrete sex hormones which play an essential role in many vital life-processes. These hormones are vital for female appeal, for the distinctive feminine appearance and the sexual urge. They vitally affect a woman's physical and mental health.

The ovaries do not actually produce ova. These eggs are produced early in a woman's life, even before her birth, in her mother's womb. They exist in latent immature form until puberty. They then begin to mature and ripen at the rate of about one a month and cause what we know as ovulation and menstruation. Scientists have found that a normal woman's ovaries contain over fifty thousand ova, or egg cells.

Every four weeks or so, an ovum matures and bursts the follicle in which it is enveloped (called the Graafian follicle). Ovulation has then occurred. The egg slowly travels toward the Fallopian tube where, if the male sperm is present, impregnation may result. Finally, the ovum makes its way into the uterus, where it gradually develops into an embryo. If more than one ovum is released at a time, twins or multiple births may follow.

FEMALE SEX HORMONES

The hormones produced by the ovaries have several vital functions. They are responsible for the development and maintenance of secondary sex characteristics. The size of breasts, the amount of pubic hair, fat deposits in the right places for typical feminine curves—all are directly affected by these female sex hormones.

There are two kinds of female sex hormones, *estrogen* and *progesterone*. Both are vital. When there is insufficient production of female sex hormones, a young girl may never acquire distinctive feminine characteristics and may actually be masculine in personality and looks. A hormone deficiency in a grown woman may cause her complexion to become flabby and wrinkled, making her look years older than her actual age.

The sex hormones have a direct effect on the proper development of external genital organs during puberty. If the ovaries are damaged in a girl, or the testes in a boy, they will remain in an infantile stage of development. The pubic hair will not grow, the breasts will not develop and the external sex organs will be underdeveloped.

Many scientists believe that aging also is tied to the hormone production of the sex glands. When the ovaries stop producing ova and sex hormone secretion diminishes or completely ceases, gradual aging sets in. However, slowdown of the sex glands can be long postponed by proper diet.

It has been found that sex glands respond to certain vitamins, especially through indirect action on the pituitary and other endocrine glands. Sufficient vitamin B_1, or thiamine, is necessary for sex hormone production. Vitamin D has been found to have a stimulating effect on the ovaries. The most important of all vitamins for your sex glands is vitamin E, particularly in pregnancy. This is the fertility vitamin. It can prevent miscarriages. It combats sterility.

It can be said that a woman is ruled by her hormones. This is particularly true when she is going through the so-called "change of life". The unpleasant features of menopause are actually symptoms of hormone starvation. A woman needs hormones to feel young and feminine, attractive and desired. Some women have lost all their sex appeal and interest in men by the time they reached their early forties. Others, well over sixty or even seventy, remain feminine and attractive to men. The difference between the groups is in their sex glands.

If you starve your glands they will age you prematurely. To retain youth and beauty you must feed your glands the nutrients they require.

HOW MRS. L. REGAINED HER YOUTH

Let me relate the case of Mrs. L., a mother of four children, whom I knew for a few years while living in Arizona. Mrs. L. was in her late thirties. She looked and felt middle-aged. Very talented and active in her youth, she had married early and spent her energy rearing four overactive boys. By the time she was thirty-five, she was exhausted. Once a fine musician, she had lost interest in music and even had to force herself to take care of her home and family.

Signs of premature aging appeared suddenly. Her hair turned gray. When she started putting on weight, her proportions changed. She acquired an old-woman look, lost her waistline. Wrinkles appeared on her face.

"I guess I'm just getting on," she said, trying to conceal her concern over her vanishing youthfulness.

For several years Mrs. L. ignored my comments on her devitalized nutrition. But after attending one of my lectures, she said to me, "I wish you could do something for me."

This was what I had been waiting for. She was now ready to assume responsibility for her condition, willing to do more than accept it without a fight.

She was far too young for a change of life. Her symptoms of premature aging were a typical case of hormone starvation. Nutritional deficiencies had caused the premature atrophy of her sex glands. Irregular and sporadic menstruations, a symptom she had neglected, indicated that she was eating too many "convenience" foods, not enough fresh fruits and mineral-rich whole grains.

I outlined a crash nutritional program for Mrs. L., featuring plenty of raw fruits and vegetables, a minimum of fat meat, but plenty of fresh, raw milk obtained from the health food store. She eliminated white sugar and white flour and all foods made with them, from her diet. She bought an electric seed grinder to make her own fresh whole wheat flour, learned to bake her own bread. She ate no more devitalized and over-refined foods such as packaged cereals, condiments, canned foods, pies or cake. I suggested that she fortify her diet with raw nuts, sunflower seeds and brewer's yeast for B-vitamins and proteins; wheat germ oil and wheat germ for vitamin E, proteins and minerals; cold pressed vegetable oils for vitamin F; rose hips for vitamin C; and two teaspoonfuls of lecithin each day. She used a natural vitamin-mineral formula and extra strong natural B-complex with B_{12} and iron; plus dessicated liver, kelp and fish liver oil for A and D. I also advised her to exercise and take long daily walks.

Mrs. L.'s transformation was miraculous. She took to her new mode of life with enthusiasm and zest, visibly growing younger with each passing week. In a few months her friends began to ask her what had happened. They hardly recognized her.

Her musical interest was reawakened. She entered the university, and graduated with a music major and started teaching music in school.

After three years on her rejuvenating diet Mrs. L. has become a totally new woman. She feels and looks younger than her age. She has acquired a youthful figure and complexion. Her menstruation cycle has become normal. She greets each day with enthusiasm. Her clothes now reflect her youthful personality. Needless to say, her husband and children are grateful for her transformation.

Mrs. L.'s case is an illustration of how revitalized glands can change your whole life. Glands can age you prematurely or keep you young far beyond middle age. The secret of youth is indeed in your glands. The hormones secreted by your sex glands are the true fountain of youth. Mrs. L. has learned that the number one factor responsible for the rejuvenation of her glandular system is nutrition. *Your glands cannot produce sufficient hormones unless they are supplied abundantly with the nutrients they need from the foods you eat.*

VITAL POINTS IN THIS CHAPTER

1. Ovaries are the female sex glands directly responsible for the healthy functioning of the reproductive and sexual system.
2. Sex hormones give you a distinctive feminine appearance, sex appeal and sexual urge. They influence the size of your breasts, regulate the fat deposits on your body and can keep you young and beautiful. Deficiencies in sex hormones can cause withered sexual ardor and premature aging.
3. How a gland-revitalizing nutritional program changed Mrs. L. from lethargic, chronically fatigued and prematurely aged woman into a young, vital and energetic wife and mother—to the delight of her husband and four children.

CHAPTER 5

MALE REPRODUCTIVE SYSTEM AND ITS FUNCTIONS

The male reproductive system like the female can be classified according to function into two groups:

1. The generative organs, *testicles* and *prostate*.
2. The copulative organ, the *penis*.

In addition, a system of *seminal ducts* connects the various sexual organs and transports the spermatozoa, prostate fluid and other secretions and hormones. The *seminal vesicles* near the prostate, produce a fluid, *semen,* which is mixed with the spermatozoa.

PENIS

Although the most important reproductive organs of the male are the testes, which produce sperm that impregnate the female egg, the *penis* is the organ designed by nature for sexual contact with the female. For semen and sperm to enter the womb, the penis must have a certain rigidity, or erection. Without sufficient erection, not only impregnation but also normal sexual intercourse is impossible. A man who is not able to achieve or sustain erection long enough to enter the vagina is termed impotent.

The erection of the male penis is directly tied with the individual's sex desires. These are triggered by erotic stimulation through imagination or sensory impressions and by the action of the hormones from the testes. If the testes are atrophied and no sex hormones are produced, erection cannot be accomplished even if erotic stimulation has occurred. Sexual desire—and consequent erection—can be stimulated by sight, smell, hearing, or by the memories connected with previous experiences. Other factors can produce an erection which has no erotic significance. Morning erections, for example, are caused by the pressure of a full bladder on the prostate gland.

WHAT CAUSES IMPOTENCE?

Given healthy, active sex glands and sufficient sexual stimulation, normal erection and normal potency should continue far into old age. But sexual power in a man is inseparably tied to his general health. The aging process greatly varies in different men. Some are biologically senile in their late thirties—some young and vital in their eighties. Healthy men have a capacity for physical love almost as long as they live.

Why then do so many men, in the prime of life and seemingly in good health, suffer from impotence or diminished sexual vigor? The answer to this question is twofold. First, the majority of all cases of impotence are psychic in origin. Second, even seemingly healthy men can have diminished sexual vigor due to undetected illness or below par condition—diabetes, inflammation of the prostate gland, hormonal deficiencies, poor nutrition, toxic influences common to modern life, such as tobacco, lead poisoning, excessive alcohol drinking, hormones residues in foods, etc. Some common causes of diminished potency are obesity, physical or mental stress and undereating, or starvation.

PROSTATE GLAND

The *prostate gland* is located just below the bladder. It encloses the neck of the urethra and is about the size of a chestnut. The prostate gland produces an alkaline fluid that is released and combined with semen. Some doctors feel this gland is not absolutely essential and that it can be removed without great threat to virility or fertility. Other researchers state that prostate secretions play an important role in the sexual act and in reproduction.

The prostate is frequently a site of acute or chronic inflammations and enlargement. Various causes have been ascribed for prostate disorders, such as a regular practice of *coitus interruptus* (withdrawal), abuse of alcohol, nutritional deficiency. We will discuss these causes in more detail in Chapter 13.

OTHER MALE SEX ORGANS

Epididymes are coiled-up tubes located above the testicles. Spermatozoa are stored in the epididymes until ready for expulsion. The *vas deferens* is a continuation of the seminal cord or duct from the epididymis to the *seminal vesicles* behind the bladder. *Cowper's glands,* tiny accessory organs, are located at the base of the penis. They manufacture a slippery fluid which lubricates the penis and the female sex organ, facilitating penetration.

THE TESTES

The *testicles* not only produce the *generative cells,* or

sperm, which perpetuate our species, but they also manufacture and secrete the male sex hormone, *testosterone,* which profoundly affects a man's sex organs, his secondary sex characteristics, his health and his state of mind.

The testicles are suspended from the groin in a sac called the scrotum, at a temperature slightly lower than normal body heat. This lower temperature may be essential for the production of sperm.

The testicles manufacture sperm. Spermatozoa are composed of an egg-shaped head and a long tail, for the mobility to reach the ovum and fertilize it. Millions of spermatozoa are released during each completed act of sexual intercourse. Only one sperm cell, the strongest and fastest, reaches the female egg.

The sperm-producing capacity of the testicles is awesome. A single emission from a normal, healthy man contains beween 400 and 500 millions of spermatozoa.

Each microscopic sperm cell contains twenty-four chromosomes, subdivided into genes, which will transmit all the hereditary characteristics of past generations.

A high-level production of sperm begins at puberty and continues until old age. Authenticated incidences have occurred where men in their eighties or even nineties have fathered children.

This colossal job, producing billions of spermatozoa throughout a man's life, is only a part of the role of the testicles. Spermatozoa production is their *exocrine* activity. Their *endocrine* activity is to manufacture the *male sex hormone, testosterone.* Exocrine hormones and secretions are sent by ducts to other parts of the body. Endocrine activity produces hormones which are absorbed by the bloodstream directly.

The testicles in men can be compared to the ovaries in women, which we have discussed in the previous chapter. The effect of the male sex hormone, testosterone, on a man's life and personality, is similar to the effect of female sex hormones on a woman.

Testosterone is responsible for the development of secondary sex characteristics at puberty, the growth of pubic hair and beard, change of voice, increase in size of the penis, and the typical masculine muscular development.

MALE SEX HORMONES

The effect of sex hormones on the life of a man is spectacular. This has been demonstrated by the effect of castration, the surgical procedure of removing the testes. The operation is frequently performed on male animals, usually to change an intractable beast into a docile one which can be used for domestic work, as in the case of oxen and horses. In other cases, castration is used to facilitate fattening.

But the most striking illustration of the effect of castration has been seen in human beings. Castration was known in ancient times in the Middle East and Europe. Eunuchs—castrated men—were employed as harem guards. At another time and in another place, they were singers in all-male choirs. Castrated before puberty, these men had no hair growth on their faces and bodies. Their torsos were effeminate and fat, their genital organs infantile, their voices high-pitched. They were docile and lazy. Naturally they had no reproductive capacities, nor did they have any sex drive.

The famous Austrian research physiologist, Professor Eugen Steinach, conducted a series of dramatic experiments on the effects of sex hormones. He de-sexed male and female animals, then transplanted female germinal glands into males and male sex glands into females. Gradually the males acquired female characteristics, including breast development. The females were masculinized by the action of male sex glands.

During the past seventy years, scientists around the world have tried to use sex glands to rejuvenate aging men and women. French scientist Edouard Brown-Sequard injected testicular extracts into both animals and men and claimed that the subjects were miraculously rejuvenated. Steinach developed what is now known as vasoligation, the tying of sperm ducts. His theory was that destroying the sperm-producing activity of the testes would stimulate their hormone-producing process. Dramatic cases of rejuvenation and renewed sexual potency—though, of course, not fertility—were reported as a result of the Steinach operations. A Russian scientist, Dr. Serge Voronoff, performed sensational testicular transplants from apes to aging men. Hundreds of operations were made and dramatic results reported. While all these attempts to rejuvenate aging bodies eventually failed, they demonstrated that youthful virility and sexual potency are dependent on the sex glands and their hormone-producing activity. The way to keep young and virile is not by replacing starved sexual glands with monkey glands, but by rejuvenating and stimulating the original glands with proper living habits and good nutrition.

Surgical rejuvenation techniques failed because they accomplished only temporary results. Vasoligation briefly stimulated the sex hormone output, but eventually caused the degeneration of the testes. Transplanted animal glands caused also only a short-lived upsurge of sexual stimulation.

NUTRITION AND SEXUAL VIRILITY

A normal functioning of the male sex glands is necessary for optimal male virility and normal sexual desires. Glands need certain proteins, vitamins, minerals and fatty acids, in order to function properly. They must draw these substances from the food we eat. Not enough scientific research has been done to point in detail the exact mechanics of this relationship between nutrition and sex glands, but sufficient information is available to indicate that *the relationship definitely exists.*

It is known that sufficient amounts of vitamins A and E

are necessary for the proper functioning of sex glands and for sufficient hormone production.[1] Drs. P. L. Harris, F. Verzar, and others, in their report to The International Congress on Vitamin E, indicated that a lack of vitamin E can cause degeneration of the testicles and diminished hormone production.[2] Also, vitamin E is anti-oxidant and therefore protects sex hormones from destruction by oxidation.

Several of the B-vitamins are essential for hormone production as well. Vitamin B_1, or thiamine, is vital to the pituitary, which in turn stimulates the sex glands. A deficiency in vitamin B_6 has caused impotence in men,[3] and deficiency of another B-vitamin, choline, has been shown to disrupt the proper balance between male and female sex hormones in the system. In the normal human body, the endocrine glands secrete both androgenic and estrogenic hormones which stimulate male and female characteristics. The liver regulates the balance between the two. A deficiency of choline, thiamine, and riboflavin (all B-vitamins) may prevent the liver from keeping the proper hormonal balance. This may lead to serious sexual disturbances in both male and female, as demonstrated by Dr. Gerson R. Biskind, of California. For example, excess of estrogenic hormones in the male may cause sterility. Protein deficiency, as well as general malnutrition, can cause sexual senility.[4] It has been observed that men in concentration camps and famine areas lose all interest in sex. On the other hand, men in Hunza and Bulgaria, two of the "healthiest" nations in the world, are reported to have fathered children after the age

---

[1] Mason, K. E., SEX AND INTERNAL SECRETIONS, Williams & Wilkins, Baltimore, 1939

[2] Harris, P. L., et al., Report to *International Congress on Vitamin E,* 1955

[3] Kinny, T. D., et al., *Journal of Exper. Medicine,* 102, 151, 1955

[4] Zubirán, S., et al., VITAMINS AND HORMONES, Academic Press, New York, 1953

of one hundred.[5] These people live on diets of wholesome natural foods, low in animal fats and rich in fruits, vegetables, whole grains, honey, milk and milk products.

If nutritional deficiencies can cause loss of virility and even impotence, why do such sexual disorders flourish in the United States, which is reputedly the best fed country in the world? The answer is simple. Although abundant food is available, many Americans—almost half, according to a report by the U.S. Department of Agriculture—suffer from nutritional deficiencies. This is partly due to devitalized and refined American food in which many vital nutrients have been destroyed, partly to widespread ignorance on which foods to eat for optimum nutrition. Many wives feed their men diets from which most of the vitamins important for virility have been removed. Vitamin E, which normally is found in whole grains and vegetable oils, is practically nonexistent in white bread and processed oils. Vitamins are largely removed or destroyed by food processing.

In Chapter 9 I will discuss optimum nutrition for sexual virility in some detail. Suffice here to say that your glands can be stimulated to a peak of their healthy power by proper nutritional habits. Foods rich in vitamins identified with sexual and reproductive functions are:

- Wheat germ oil, wheat germ, cold-pressed vegetable oils and whole grain products for vitamins E, B, proteins and essential fatty acids.
- Green and bright-colored vegetables and fish liver oil for vitamin A, and
- Brewer's yeast, liver, whole grain products, raw nuts and seeds, milk and milk products for B-complex vitamins, minerals, and proteins.

[5] Taylor, A., HUNZA HEALTH SECRETS, Prentice-Hall, Inglewood Cliffs, N. J., 1964

VITAL POINTS IN THIS CHAPTER

1. Sex hormones produced by the male sex glands have a spectacular effect on man's life and personality.

2. Although the majority of cases of male impotence are psychic in origin, many are organic. Irrational diet, smoking, excessive drinking, poisons in food and environment, use of drugs and nutritional deficiencies can all cause diminution of male virility and potency.

3. A plentiful production of sex hormones is essential for the maximum of masculine power.

4. Glandular activity and hormone production can be favorably affected by proper nutrition.

CHAPTER 6

IS NUTRITION THE WHOLE ANSWER?

THE UNEQIVOCAL ANSWER to the title above is: of course not. Nutrition is singularly the most important factor affecting one's health. And unless you are in reasonably good health you cannot enjoy adequate and satisfactory sexual relations. This is only common sense.

But, as important as nutrition obviously is for man's sexual life, it is not the whole answer. Man's sexual activity, perhaps more than any other phase of his life, is affected by his psyche. Inhibitions, fears, even boredom, can retard man's sexual life and make enjoyable sexual expression impossible. It is estimated by most authorities that ninety percent of all male impotence has a psychological origin.

One of the most common causes of impotence is fear—fear of being unable to achieve erection, fear of inadequacy. One or two unsuccessful experiences may establish a feeling of inferiority, a subconscious belief that failure will happen again. The mechanics of our minds are such that we bring about the negative results which we fear. Failure creates failure, just as success creates success.

Another frequent cause of impotence is ignorance. Ignorance is perhaps the greatest single cause of sexual unhappiness and broken marriage. Fears of adverse results of childhood masturbation are a case in point. Lives have been totally ruined, not because of the results of masturbation, but because of fear in the minds of those who practiced it. They had heard it would cause irrevocable damage to their minds and bodies. In part the blame for such ungrounded belief must be placed upon early medical writers who linked excessive childhood masturbation with all kinds of pathological development, including insanity. It has been known for several decades and reported in medical literature and sex education books that such fears are *totally ungrounded*. This conclusion is based on a number of scientific studies. Masturbation is not more injurious than a normal sexual act. Kinsey studies revealed that an overwhelming majority of all men have masturbated at some time in their lives. But such reports are not read by all, and the scientific facts are not as well known as they should be.

Other fears and feelings of inferiority may be in regard to the size of the penis or to the frequency of intercourse. Here again some of the old erotic books and stories have accomplished more harm than good. The belief that only a large male member can give sexual satisfaction is totally ungrounded and disproved by medical research. More than anywhere else, the quality, not the quantity is what counts here. Furthermore, actual variations in penis size of healthy men are extremely insignificant. In erection there is little difference, as demonstrated by actual measurements made in various countries. In a flaccid condition there may be considerable variation in size. In any event, the small difference in size is not a factor in successful intercourse and sexual enjoyment.

In regard to the frequency of intercourse, many men suffer feelings of inferiority after reading wild stories and hearing tales of marathon sex races. The frequency of sexual activity varies considerably in the same individual at different periods of his life. Naturally, sex is more frequent in the twenties than in the sixties. Also, much depends on the amount of interest and energy one is allocating to sexual matters. A serious preoccupation with strenuous physical or mental work, for example, will result in a diminished amorous interest. A mathematician, preoccupied with solving complicated calculus problems, is not an urgent lover—neither is a laborer digging ditches from morning to evening on meager fare. On the other hand, the same individuals in the relaxed atmosphere of a seashore holiday, free from worries and responsibilities, can surprise themselves and their wives with their virile playboy qualities.

"An impotent man around the house is as great a reflection on his wife as dirty floors or unmade beds, and far commoner," says Dr. George Belham, a famous authority on sexology.[1] A woman who is domineering, disrespectful, demanding, nagging, critical, who fails to keep herself tidy, attractive and desirable, and who takes her man's marital responsibilities for granted, will eventually destroy her husband's libido and make him impotent long before he reaches middle age. An intelligent, wise woman can maintain and bolster a man's libido by making him feel important, capable, admired and loved.

Boredom is one of the common reasons for loss of sexual sparkle, especially in older married couples. The same routine, the same positions year-after-year-after-year, in the same place, the same time, can kill anybody's amorous desires. Sex requires constant exploration for new forms of expression. Or it will become routine.

Unfortunately, we are held back and are afraid to do "what comes naturally." We have been brainwashed

---

[1] Belham, George, THE VIRILITY DIET, Dell Publishing Co., Inc., New York, 1968. Copyright (c) 1965 by George Belham.

from our childhood to consider certain ways or positions for sexual expression as proper and "normal" and some others as "abnormal." Our joyous sexual expression is thwarted by incorrect ideas and Victorian taboos. Happily, books in growing number now offer frank education to couples who want to rejuvenate and revitalize their sex lives.

To achieve full sexual enjoyment, inhibitions, imagined fears and inferiority feelings must be corrected. If your sexual life is retarded through psychological causes, improved nutrition probably will do you little good. You should go to an experienced psychiatrist or marriage counselor and untangle your anxieties. Also, if you suffer from ill health, your sexual relations may suffer, too. If you are always tired, have little interest in work or play, suffer from lack of appetite—see your doctor. These may be only minor symptoms, easily wiped out by rest and improved nutrition. Or, they may require a doctor's urgent attention.

The scope of this study is limited to the nutritional aspects of sex. A danger exists, because of this limitation, that the reader will be impressed with the importance of nutrition and will forget the other factors involved.

I do, however, want to point out that with all my enthusiasm for nutrition I do not intend to minimize the importance of psychological and sociological factors in sexual health. An improved nutritional status *may help* an individual to cope even with his emotional problems, but food alone cannot eliminate feelings of unworthiness, inferiority and rejection. Such feelings are deep-rooted, often stemming from ego-damaging experiences in childhood. The best means of correcting these emotional problems—perhaps with the help of a psychoanalyst—is to place them in their proper light. Once understanding is established, restoration of confidence and ability will soon follow.

On the other hand, when nutritional deficiencies have been a contributing cause of sexual disturbance, improved nutrition can have a dramatic effect. Restored glandular activity will not only affect the physical well-being of the individual but also his mental health, his emotional feelings, his desires and urges. Optimum nutrition can indeed be a solid base for better physical health, as well as for more emotional stability.

VITAL POINTS IN THIS CHAPTER

1. Although many reproductive disorders and sexual inadequacies are nutritional in origin, nutrition is not the whole answer to complex sexual problems.
2. Most cases of male impotence have non-organic causes—inhibitions, fears, ignorance, boredom.
3. The psychic causes of sexual disorders and impotence must be corrected before the full benefits of revitalizing nutrition can be realized.

CHAPTER 7

"SINCE THE BEGINNING OF TIME . . ."

SINCE THE BEGINNING of time, at least time as we have recorded it, men have sought ways of prolonging or increasing sexual vigor. Young men have searched for greater ecstasy and older men have fought the onset of sexual decline. This interest has not been limited to men only. Women have sought means of heightening their sexual enjoyment and, an important goal in past ages, of avoiding the stigma of barrenness.

This preoccupation with sexual virility and reproductive capacity is as universal as it is natural. The modern sciences of psychoanalysis and psychosomatic medicine have demonstrated that man's total self-esteem, self-confidence and emotional stability are linked with his sexual self-confidence. The loss of sexual virility, organic or imaginary, can severely damage man's emotional health and shake the balance of his personality. Man's need for sexual self-esteem is as strong as his need for physical satisfaction. To be sexually competent equates with success. Incompetence has been cause for shame. Thus, it is easy to understand why throughout the ages men have been concerned with their sexual health and have sought means of preserving—or recovering—sexual vigor.

APHRODISIACS—WHAT THEY ARE

The dictionary defines an aphrodisiac as a food or drug that arouses sexual desire. Many of those used in the past were harmful to health. Medical writings of those periods contain numerous reports of damaged health and even deaths as a result of toxic aphrodisiacs. Early man had a phallic approach to virility and considered that the source of sexual power was in the penis itself. He therefore employed various external applications directly on the penis to cause erection. Many of the remedies used for this purpose were highly irritable—for instance, burning nettles and hot peppers. Ancient manuals list various ointments for topical application. Invariably these were made of strong herbs and chemical substances more likely to cause inflammations than joyous erection.

Some drugs used as aphrodisiacs over the ages were so toxic that in many cases they proved fatal. The notorious *Spanish fly* was popular during the Middle Ages in Italy, France and the Arab countries. Its popularity has survived in some areas. Cantharides—Spanish fly preparations—still are offered for sale in some border towns. Spanish fly is obtained from beetles. Taken internally, it produces a violent irritation in the intestines, kidneys and generative organs. Spanish fly causes an erection due to swelling, inflammation and congestion as a reaction to its toxic action. It often damages the kidneys. Dr. George Belham tells of a banquet where cantharides were mixed in a special spice. Guests used the spice in large quantities with every dish. The next morning all who had used the spice were dead, "unfortunately without leaving any indication as to whether it had proved effective during the night," adds Dr. Belham.[1]

---

[1] Belham, George, THE VIRILITY DIET, Dell Publishing Co., Inc., New York, 1968. Copyright (c) 1965 by George Belham.

Strychnine, a highly poisonous crystalline alkaloid, was another common toxic drug used for aphrodisiac effect. In very small doses, strychnine stimulates the nervous system and may alert the senses. Larger amounts may cause severe convulsions or death.

TRUE AND FALSE APHRODISIACS

People of the past, in their desire to restore amatory prowess, resorted to anything that promised a quick effect. Our forefathers did not know why certain foods, plants or drugs acted as they did. People knew little about nutrition and the inner workings of the reproductive system. Even if some of the foods and plants they used can now be justified pharmacologically and nutritionally as conducive to greater virility, the difference between safety and toxicity was not well known.

With our present knowledge of nutrition and medicine, we have no excuse for using toxic psuedo-aphrodisiacs. We do not approve or recommend any artificial stimulants, nor do we subscribe to the idea that sexual desire should be stimulated beyond the normal. Artificial stimulation will gradually result in a total loss of sexual desire and potency. Stimulating an interest in sex for sex's sake, pleasure for pleasure's sake, or for bedroom championship, is not a purpose of this work. Sex and sex happiness are important, indeed, but only in the frame of the overall health picture; as a part of the total emotional, physical and spiritual development of the individual.

Admittedly, there is no simple cure for impotence. No single drug or food by itself is a cure for impotence. But it is equally true that optimum nutrition and proper diet are the ultimate secret for optimum health and sexual virility.

Dr. George Belham states: "Sexual activity is one of the most sensitive and easily disturbed bodily functions, and it is the first to be affected by unhealthy eating."[1] When sexual activity is disturbed and virility is lowered due to "unhealthy eating," corrected nutritional patterns and special dietary additions can do miracles in restoring sexual health and libido. It is from this nutritional angle that we are interested in the so-called aphrodisiacs. The only aphrodisiacs advocated in this book are natural, completely harmless foods and food substances. These foods do not cause artificial stimulation on sexual centers and reproductive organs. They act entirely by virtue of the nutritional properties they contain. Their virility-restorative property is in feeding nutrition-starved endocrine glands and stimulating hormone production.

Our view on aphrodisiacs can be summarized as follows:

1. All artificial stimulants of sexual desire, and all drugs and topical applications aimed at effecting erection by causing irritation of the generative organs, are potentially harmful and their use is definitely not recommended.
2. Where a diminished sexual interest is due to physical weakness, poor health, hormone inadequacies and glandular disorders, improved nutrition and special virility foods can favorably affect health and bring about improved sexual activity.

In the following review of ancient medical writings and erotic discourses, we have left out anything that has anything to do with harmful, artificial stimulants. Likewise, we have left out all worthless magic customs and remedies.

Our study of ancient writings is limited to various foods and food substances used and recommended for centuries. Many have been confirmed by recent medical research as having real value—others are still "unproven," except for the fact that they have been faithfully used for hundreds of years, which, according to some authorities, *is* proof of their efficiency.

ASIA—THE CENTER OF THE ART AND THE SCIENCE OF LOVE

Asians always regarded sex as an art to be studied, learned, and perfected. The greatest writers, historians, and physicians of Asian history were preoccupied with erotic subjects and with the search for aphrodisiacs, as much ancient literature will testify.

INDIA

Of all the Oriental countries, India is perhaps the most sex-conscious. In Indian writings, Kama—the love pleasure—is the greatest virtue and joy of life. The Hindu is basically a vegetarian and his dietary aphrodisiacs are naturally centered around foods of vegetable origin. An Indian believes that the woman is an equal in sexual intercourse; that man's success as a lover is largely dependent on a cooperative and skillful partner. The Indian woman is trained in the intricate art of aphrodisiac cooking to help her man achieve the peak of his sexual power. The emphasis is on a wealth of native herbs and spices. Most Indian recipes name garlic, onions, leeks and beans as foods of special aphrodisiac value. Garlic was especially held in esteem. The Indian national favorites—curry, rice, chutney, mango and ghee—were also claimed to give exceptional sexual powers.

The KAMA SUTRA of Vatsyayana Malanaga names several foods as means of increasing sexual vigor. The most often named are milk, sugar, honey, ghee (melted butter), eggs, sesame seeds, wheat and beans.

Here are a few samples:

- "A man obtains sexual vigor by drinking milk mixed with sugar, the root of the uchchata plant, the piper chaba, and liquorice."

• "Drinking milk with sugar, and having the testicle of a ram or a goat boiled in it, is also productive of vigor . . ."

• "In the same way, if a man mixes with rice the eggs of a sparrow, and having boiled this in milk, adds to it ghee and honey, and drinks of it as much as necessary, this will produce the same effect."

• "If a man takes the outer coverings of sesamum seeds, and soaks them with the eggs of sparrows, and then, having boiled them in milk, mixed with sugar and ghee, along with the fruits of the trapa bispinosa and the kasurika plant, and adding to it the flour of wheat and beans, and then drinks of this composition, he is said to be able to enjoy many women."

• "If ghee, honey, sugar and liquorice in equal quantities, the juice of the fennel plant, and milk are mixed together, this nectar-like composition is said to be holy, and provocative of sexual vigor, a preservative of life, and sweet to the taste."

Another Indian book, ANANGA-RANGA, or Hindu Art of Love, gives the following receipes to restore potency and excite desire:[2]

• "Expose the juice of bhuya-kokali (solanum jacquini) under the heat of the sun until it dries and then mix it with clarified butter, candied sugar, and honey. This preparation gives the strength of ten men, and enables but one man to satisfy ten women."

• Take the outside covering of the anvalli, (an astringent nut) extract its juice and expose this under the sun until dry. After this it should be mixed with powder from the same tree, and, before congress, eaten with clarified but-

---

[2] Walton, Alan Hull, APHRODISIACS FROM LEGEND TO PRESCRIPTION, Associated Booksellers, Bridgeport, Conn. 06606. The quote is Alan H. Walton's translation from the French edition of ANANGA-RANGA: TRAITE HINDOU DE l'AMOUR CONJUGAL, Bibliothèque des Curieux, Paris, 1910

ter, candied sugar and honey. From this results a prodigious development of the genital; even an old man becomes like a young one.

In addition to the often mentioned milk, honey, sugar (raw, unrefined sugar, of course), ghee (liquified butter), and various spices, wild rice mixed with honey is also mentioned.

CHINA AND JAPAN

In China and Japan aphrodisiac cookery has been popular throughout history, but the recipes have been published only rarely; they are usually shrouded in secrecy and passed down from father to son.

One of the most famous—and most powerful—Chinese aphrodisiacs is *Bird Nest Soup.* A noted scholar on aphrodisiacs, Alan Hull Walton, says that "the aphrodisiac effect of bird nest soup cannot be denied."[2] Bird nest soup is prepared from the nest of the sea-swallow. And here is the secret of its aphrodisiac efficacy—sea-swallows make their nests from seaweed plants which they glue together with fish spawn. Seaweed is, of course, one of the wonder-foods of nature, the powerful storehouse of important minerals, particularly iodine which is so essential for the health of the endocrine glands, specifically the thyroid. An iodine deficiency can cause goiter and disrupt the normal functions of the thyroid gland. Thyroid is of special importance to the sex drive. An underactive thyroid can diminish your desire and cause impotence. Kelp (seaweed) is the richest natural source of iodine and other vital minerals, such as magnesium, sodium and potassium. Seaweed is used extensively in Oriental cooking, especially in Japan.

The other ingredient of bird nest soup is fish spawn. Spawn is, of course, fish eggs, and is known to be abundant in many nutritive factors, particularly in the mineral *phos-*

phorus. Alan Hull Walton suggests that phosphorus is a powerful aphrodisiac substance, "increasing both desire and erection."[2]

In bird nest soup we see a typical example of an "old wives' tale" turned into a scientifically confirmed fact. Much in ancient aphrodisiac lore is pure nonsense and superstition. But now and then you will find a valuable food or substance that the ancients discovered empirically. Bird nest soup seems to be one such aphrodisiac which can be pharmacologically and nutritionally explained and justified.

Two other popular Chinese aphrodisiacs are *ginger* (also used in India, Turkey, and Arabian countries) and *ginseng root.* Ginseng root, which resembles the human figure, is used widely in the Orient as a general tonic. It is credited with many remarkable health-giving properties and also with an aphrodisiac effect. Ginseng has survived the test of use for thousands of years. Health magazines in the United States and Europe still advertise tonics made with it. What factor accounts for its professed properties is unknown. According to a U.S. Public Health Service report, an analysis of ginseng failed to find any pharmacological reason for the root's reputed effects. Some scientists believe that the ginseng's resemblance to the human figure has a psychological influence on those who believe in it. Whatever the true facts, millions of people, both in the Orient and the Western world, continue to use ginseng and are satisfied with the imagined or real benefits they derive from it.

Garlic, onions, bamboo shoots and sea foods are other aphrodisiac foods used by the Chinese. Also considered aphrodisiac is Nuoc-man, a spicy sauce, rich in fish oils and phosphorus.

ARABIAN COUNTRIES

One of the most famous amatory works from Arab countries is THE PERFUMED GARDEN OF THE SHEIKH NEFZAOUI, a manual of Arabian erotology and sexology. Some doctors and sexologists consider The Perfumed Garden a significant study. In the words of Dr. Franklin S. Klaf, M.D., it is "an important document in the history of ideas . . . ."

The Perfumed Garden was written in the fourteenth century and first translated from Arabic to French in 1850. The first English translation was made from the French by Sir Richard Burton and published in 1886. The quotations used here are taken from the recent edition published by Lancer Books, Inc., New York, which used the original translation made for the Kama Shastra Society of London and Benares in the early 1800's.

The Perfumed Garden is a detailed manual on coital techniques, treatment of impotence and female sterility, dimensions of the male and female sexual organs and various means of increasing virility; in general, it is filled with advice on "everything favorable to coition." The Perfumed Garden also contains a great amount of advice on aphrodisiacs. For the purpose of this work we are interested only in the chapters dealing with aphrodisiac foods and drinks.[3]

First, the Sheikh Nefzaoui has no ifs or buts as to the direct relationship between nutrition and sex. He states with unqualified certainty that not only general health but also sexual power and virility depend on good nutrition:

"On the other hand, the condition of the body, and consequently the quality of the sperm, depends directly upon the food you take. If, therefore, a man will passionately give himself up to the enjoyment of coition, without undergoing too great fatigue, he must live upon strengthening food . . ."

The "strengthening foods" listed for this purpose are

---

[3] THE PERFUMED GARDEN of the Sheikh Nefzaoui, Lancer Books, Inc., New York, 1968

"exciting comfits" (dishes prepared from fresh fruits and honey), aromatic plants (vegetables and herbs), meats, honey, eggs, and "other similar viands."

In Chapter XX, The Sheikh Nefzaoui goes into detailed instructions and recipes for these "strengthening foods."

> "Know, O Visir (God be good to you) that this chapter contains the most useful instructions—how to increase the intensity of the coitus—and that the latter part is profitable to read for an old as well as for the man in his best years and for the young man.
>
> "He who makes it a practice to eat every day fasting the yolks of eggs, without the white part, will find in this ailment an energetic stimulant for the coitus. The same is the case with the man who during three days eats of the same mixed with onions.
>
> "He who boils asparagus, and then fries them in fat, and then pours upon them the yolks of eggs with pounded condiments and eats every day of this dish, will grow very strong for the coitus, and find in it a stimulant for his amorous desires.
>
> "He who peels onions, puts them into a saucepan, with condiments and aromatic substances, and fries the mixture with oil and yolks of eggs, will acquire a surpassing and invaluable vigor for the coitus, if he will partake of dish for several days.
>
> "Camel's milk mixed with honey and taken regularly developes a vigor for copulation . . . and causes the virile member to be on the alert night and day."

Eggs, milk, and honey come forth in practically every recipe as potent active ingredients. Here is a recipe recommended for those who wish to acquire a peak of sexual vigor:

> "He must get a great number of eggs, so that he may eat to surfeit, and fry them with fresh fat and butter: when done he immerses them in honey working

> the whole mass well together. He must eat of them as much as possible with little bread, and he may be certain that for the whole night his member will not give him any rest."

Nuts as aphrodisiac food are also mentioned in THE PERFUMED GARDEN.

> "He who feels that he is weak for coition should drink before going to bed a glassful of very thick honey and eat twenty almonds and one hundred grains of the pine tree. He must follow this *regime* for three days. He may also pound onion seeds, sift it and mix it afterwards with honey, stirring the mixture well, and taking of this mixture while still fasting."

Aphrodisiac beverages recommended by Sheikh are based on the same basic ingredients: honey and onions. Here is a recipe for a drink that is promised to "give vigor for coition":

> "Take one part of the juice pressed out of pounded onions, and mix it with two parts of purified honey. Heat the mixture over a fire until the onion juice has disappeared and the honey only remains. Then take the residue from the fire, let it cool, and preserve it for use when wanted. Then mix of the same one part with three parts of water and let chick-peas be macerated in this fluid for one day and one night.
>
> "This beverage is to be partaken of during winter and on going to bed. Only a small quantity is to be taken, and only for one day. The member of him who has drunk of it will not give him much rest during the night that follows. . . ."

THE PERFUMED GARDEN was written long before modern methods of chemical analysis were discovered. The author, who unquestionably was much before his time and had a good understanding of the psychological and physiological aspects of sex, could not know the nutritional reasons for many of his aphrodisiac recipes. Their popularity was based on empirical evidence, or the test of time. Many of the foods recommended in THE PERFUMED·GARDEN, such as milk, honey, eggs, onions and nuts, have not only survived the test of time until the present generation, but have now been scientifically proven valuable for general health. As we will see in Chapter 11, these foods can indeed spark your sexual desires and increase your virility.

Finally, Sheikh Nefzaoui gives the following advice in regard to health, nutrition and sex:

> "Know that there are eight things which give strength. . . These are: bodily health, the absence of all care and worry, an unembarrassed mind, natural gaiety of the spirit, good nourishment, wealth, the variety of the faces of women and the variety of their complexions . . ."
>
> "A robust constitution is indispensible for copulation, and he who is endowed with it may give himself up to pleasure without danger . . ."

> "Eat slowly, if your food shall do you good,
> And take good care, that it be well digested.
> Beware of things which want hard mastication;
> They are bad nourishment, so keep from them.
> Drink not directly after finishing your meal,
> Or else you go half way to meet an illness.
> Keep not within you what is of excess,
> And if you were in most susceptible circles,
> Attend to this well before seeking your bed,
> For rest this is the first necessity.
> From medicines and drugs keep well away,
> And do not use them unless very ill . . ." [3])

EUROPE AND MIDDLE EAST

The oldest reference to food with aphrodisiac properties

is found in the Bible. Genesis 30, 14-17 tells of *mandrake,* a plant of the potato family, which was valued by the Jews as possessing the property to stimulate potency and increase fertility.

> "And Reuben went in the days of wheat harvest, and found mandrakes in the field, and brought them into his mother Leah. Then Rachel said to Leah, Give me, I pray thee, of thy son's mandrakes.
>
> "And she said unto her, Is it a small matter that thou hast taken my husband? and wouldest thou take away my son's mandrakes also? And Rachel said, Therefore he shall lie with thee tonight for thy son's mandrakes.
>
> "And Jacob came out of the field in the evening, and Leah went out to meet him, and said, Thou must come in unto me; for surely I have hired thee with my son's mandrakes. And he lay with her that night.
>
> "And God hearkened unto Leah, and she conceived, and bare Jacob the fifth son."

Ancient Greece and Rome also valued mandrake, as writings of such authorities as Pliny and Dioscorides show. Phythagoras and Plutarch knew about it. Many ancient writers refer to mandrake and claim that not only does it increase male sexual desire and potency, but it is also a remedy for female sterility.

Actually, mandrake is of the same plant family as Chinese ginseng, mentioned earlier in this chapter. Both are roots with resemblance to the human form.

Another well-known aphrodisiac plant used widely by Greeks and Romans was *satyrion,* the root of the male orchid, *Orchis mascula.* The root was dissolved in goat's milk and was claimed to "rekindle the fires of love in exhausted old men."

Greek erotic writings frequently mention eggs, onions, beans, honey and all kinds of shellfish and snails. The reputation of shellfish and snails continues—snails have been the most popular aphrodisiac food in France in modern times. Fish and oysters were considered potent aphrodisiacs throughout the ages.

Today we know that fish, particularly oysters, abound in phosphorus, zinc and vitamins.

It is noteworthy that animal meat, looked upon today by many as a source of virility, was not regarded by the ancients as such; although the testes of all animals, especially those of the ram, ass, or lion, were believed to be potent foods.

Many vegetables, plants, seeds, nuts and herbs are frequently mentioned, such as onions, garlic, cabbage, asparagus, peas, almonds, sesame seeds, cucumber and mushrooms. Fruits are conspicuously absent from the list of foods recommended for virility by the ancients, with one exception —the apple. In ancient Greece and Rome the apple was considered a symbol of life. Old Scandinavian legends tell that the gods, when they grew old and needed rejuvenation, would feast on a diet of apples.

PREMATURE EJACULATION AND THE "STAYING POWER"

Man's sexual capacity is not measured only by the quantity but also by the quality of his sexual performance. To a great extent, his sexual capacity is determined by his ability to control himself and regulate the male orgasm and the length of intercourse. The problem of premature ejaculation is a real one for a great number of men, who are sexually potent otherwise. Every normal man experiences premature ejaculation occasionally. This can be caused by prolonged abstinence or pronounced anxiety and tension, fear or fatigue. If this happens only occasionally, it should not be a cause for concern. But if the premature ejaculation becomes a habit, it may ruin sexual enjoyment of both partners.

Premature ejaculations can have many causes; by far the majority of them are mental. The usual treatment advocated by most sexologists and marriage counselors would be the control of emotions during the sexual act. When you feel that you are about to climax, slow down or stop motions and force yourself to think of something unrelated to sex, something of interest to you—for example, news of the day, or important business dealings. This will dampen your sexual excitement, prevent premature ejaculation and make prolongation of intercourse possible.

The ancient erotic writings, although recognizing the importance of a proper mental attitude, also prescribed certain nutritional means of preventing premature ejaculation and increasing the "staying power."

In The Perfumed Garden, the Sheikh Nefzaoui writes:

> "The man whose ejaculation is too precipitate must take nutmeg and incense (oliban) mixed together with honey."

Sir Richard Burton, in his Arabian Nights, writes:

> ". . . Eastern books on domestic medicine consist mostly of two parts: the first of general prescriptions, and the second of aphrodisiacs, especially of those *que prolongent le plaisir*. . . The essence of the "retaining art" is to avoid over-tension of the muscles and to preoccupy the brain: hence in coition Hindus will drink sherbert, chew betelnut, and even smoke."

More recently, the English beers (either "bitter" or "mild") have been reputed to aid the prolongation of coitus.[2] Allan Hull Walton comments on this supposed virtue of beer that small quantities of alcohol promote muscular relaxation, remove inhibitions, and "produce in the drinker a carefree state of mind." These virtues of beer may explain its supposed efficacy in aiding cases of premature ejaculation.

ANCIENT APHRODISIACS IN THE LIGHT OF MODERN SCIENCE

The urge to restore waning sex powers has been going on

as long as man has lived. Every nation, every race and every tribe had its own favorite foods, herbs and medicines which were used for this purpose. Some of these formulas were ridiculous and would certainly not be justified in the light of modern science. Some were extremely dangeous. The famed Roman poet, Lucretius, died of one of these "love potions." Some of the recipes were based on magic. No wonder modern medical science once rejected all claims that a relationship exists between foods and physical capacity for love.

Yet many of the ancient love potions and aphrodisiac foods read conspicuously like a modern textbook on good nutrition. Honey, milk, eggs, seafoods, seaweed, nuts, sesame seeds, garlic and onions—all are high on the list recommended by modern nutrition. What seemed ridiculous to science a few decades ago, now can be backed up with newer scientific knowledge.

Official medical science would deny that any singular food or food substance can possess a mysterious potency-restoring property; but it would agree that good nutrition can have a favorable effect on a man's sexual vigor. The secret foods used by ancients and handed down from father to son (or from mother to daughter) for countless generations, may not have such miraculous effects on man's virility as ancient writings profess. Most of them, however, are certainly potent nutritious foods, which can do nothing but good for the health generally and for sexual health in particular.

Here are a few examples:

- *Milk* (and particularly goat's milk) contains *the highest grade of protein known to man.* It is more easily digested, more effectively utilized, than any other form of protein. Complete proteins of the highest possible quality are essential for the healthy functioning of endocrine and sex glands.
- *Egg yolks* contain huge amounts of licithin, a vitally important substance for the peak activity of sex glands. Lecithin is needed in great quantity for the production of sex hormones and sperm.

• *Sesame seeds* have been found abundant in important minerals, protein, lecithin and vitamins—all vital for the health of the reproductive system.

• *Honey* is a rich source of aspartic acid, the ingredient used by some modern doctors to treat female "bedroom fatigue." Honey sugars are in a pre-digested, quickly assimilable form. Sugar is important for the manufacture of male seminal fluid.

• *Oysters, nuts and pumpkin seeds* are rich sources of zinc, which has clinically been demonstrated to affect the health of the prostate and hormone-producing sex glands.

Modern science is not eager to talk about aphrodisiacs. Science does not believe that healthy sexual activity needs artificial stimulation. But feeding endocrine and sex glands properly and thus helping them to reach a peak of *healthy activity* is quite a different matter. Therefore, we like to talk of foods that spark sexual desire and increase sexual power *not as aphrodisiacs* but as *sources of nutrients* needed for the healthy function of reproductive organs and sex glands.

CHAPTER SUMMARY

1. Man has sought ways and means to prolong or increase his sexual vigor as long as he has lived, "since the beginning of time".

2. Every nation, race and tribe had its favorite aphrodisiacs—foods and formulae used to preserve or increase man's sexual power.

3. Many drugs, hallucinogens and narcotics, including alcohol, used for the purpose of arousing sexual desires, are extremely harmful substances and actually useless as aphrodisiacs, since ultimately they result in damaged health and lowered virility.

4. Many of the foods and food substances used by

ancients—Indians, Chinese, Arabs, Jews, Romans and Greeks—are potent health-giving foods which, according to modern nutritionists, have a beneficial effect on health in general, and on the healthy function of the reproductive system in particular. Such foods as honey, milk, eggs, sesame seeds, nuts, garlic, onions and seawood are gold mones of nutrients which are essential for increased vigor and sustained sexual virility.

CHAPTER 8

HIGH-PROTEIN DIET AND SEX

YOU CAN OPEN almost any popular American health book and find an exhortation common to all of them—*more, more and more protein!* Health writers and authorities may teach completely different ways to glorious health, but all agree on one point—you need lots of protein for your health.

We are brainwashed with this high-protein idea from cradle to grave, so to speak. Children are taught it in kindergarten and high school home-ec classes. The nutrition departments of our universities subscribe to it. You read it in popular magazines and the syndicated health columns of your daily newspaper. You are bombarded with high-protein propaganda from every possible direction, including roadside billboards. You are advised to eat as much protein food—meat, fish, eggs and milk—as possible. In fact, you are told that you never can have too much protein.

The twentieth century has been given many descriptive and timely names. My humble contribution to the long line of epithets includes: "The matriarchal era," "The adulation-of-youth age," "The century of chemical assault on man's environment," "The epoch of misguided scientific progress," and "The slow-extinction-through-chemistry era." But perhaps the most appropriate designation of all for the health-conscious twentieth century would be: "The era of the high-protein cult."

The high-protein dogma is so permanently engraved in our thinking that I hesitate to suggest it may be erroneous. Yet, a desire to help the sincere seeker of truth compels me to try.

"HIGH-PROTEIN CRAZE" AND HOW IT ORIGINATED

It is not difficult to understand how the high-protein myth originated. Proteins are important nutritive factors. However, Dr. Karl-Otto Aly, M.D., speaks of "the American high-protein craze," as an overemphasis placed on high-protein requirement.

Your body is built largely of proteins. Your muscles, hair, skin, vital organs and glands, even your hormones, are made of protein. Twenty per cent or more of the cell composition in your body is protein. Since your body is constantly renewing and repairing itself, you need lots of proteins in your diet for the building of new cells.

But how much is "lots?" Many experts suggest that you need from seventy to two hundred fifty grams, or even more, each day.

Scientists around the world are beginning to suspect a mistake in their estimates of our protein needs. More and more evidence is turning up to show that enough protein is good, but too much is bad. Sugar is essential for our health. But too much sugar in the diet has been established as the cause of many health disorders. We need fats. But too much fat in the diet will cause a legion of troubles. Even too much of certain vitamins or minerals may cause ill health. And so it is also with proteins. As essential and important as they are, too much protein, especially cooked animal protein, may cause disordered metabolism and biochemical imbalance in the tissues, which may lead to the most common degenerative diseases, including arthritis,[1] arteriosclerosis and heart disease.[2]

WHAT ARE PROTEINS

Proteins are molecules composed of thousands of smaller particles called amino acids. There are over twenty known amino acids; ten of these are considered essential, because the body cannot manufacture them within the system and they must be supplied by the food you eat.

Every part of your body is built of different amino acids and their combinations. When you eat proteins, the protein molecules are broken down into separate amino acids during the digestive process; then they are absorbed by the bloodstream. Every cell of your body selects the amino acids it needs from the blood plasma.

Not all foods contain all the amino acids, although almost all natural foods contain some proteins. Foods that contain all the essential amino acids are called complete protein foods. Meat, fish, eggs, milk, and cheese and such vegetable sources as soy beans, sesame seeds, some nuts, potatoes and most green vegetables, contain complete proteins. Most grains and beans are deficient in some of the essential amino acids although in combination with foods that do contain the missing amino acids, they become valuable protein foods.

---

[1] The American Medical Association News Release, June 21, 1965

[2] Gerber, Donald A., Professor of medicine at N. Y. State University, report at the Annual Rheumatism Foundation meeting, New York Times, April 7, 1965

HOW MUCH PROTEIN DO WE ACTUALLY NEED?

Studies made by such well-known authorities on nutrition as Drs. Ragnar Berg, William C. Rose, V. O. Sivén, D. M. Hegsted, and R. Chittenden, show that our actual daily requirement of protein is somewhere between thirty and forty grams. More recent studies made by German professor K. Eimer and Japanese scientist Dr. M. Kuratsune, support this estimation. One of the most reliable sources on matters of nutrition today is The International Society for Research on Nutrition and Vital Substances, the Scientific Council of which is comprised of four hundred doctors of medicine, biochemistry, nutrition and natural sciences. This foremost scientific authority has stated that our "classical" protein-requirement tables need an overhaul. The basis of a diet which assures a healthy and well-balanced nutrition should consist of whole cereal products, milk and milk products and fresh vegetables and fruits. "Meat, fish, and eggs can supplement this basic diet, but *a daily intake of these foods is not necessary*," says The International Society for Research on Nutrition and Vital Substances.

The outdated calculations in regard to protein need were based on nineteenth century research by Justus von Liebig, Karl von Voit and Max Rubner, who believed that man's daily need of protein was one hundred twenty grams. Until today many of the beliefs and the opinions regarding protein need were based on these men's faulty calculations. As Dr. H. B. Lewis has pointed out, it is indeed "very dangerous when great men make mistakes." Although the official tables of protein need have been slowly going down for the last several decades, and are now set at about one-half gram per pound per day of body weight, many authorities continue to cling to the old, outdated "more-more-and more protein" idea, with emphasis on animal protein.

In accord with the latest research, and taking into consideration the great variation in protein need of each individual and the extra demands in conditions of stress, a generous conclusion would be that 50 to 60 grams a day of protein, *derived 75 to 80 percent from vegetable sources,* is sufficient for optimum health. Proteins in excess of this amount are *not needed by the body and are only burned as fuel for energy. As fuel, proteins are inferior to natural carbohydrates and fats.*

FADS AND FALLACIES ABOUT PROTEIN

1. *"YOU NEED MEAT FOR PROTEINS!"* This is one of the most common fallacies which is best disproved by the following facts. About half of the world population do not eat meat for religious or other reasons. There are also large groups of people in the United States, such as Seventh-Day Adventists, who do not eat meat all—and display much better health than the average American: 40 percent less heart disease, 1000 percent less lung cancer, and 100 percent lower total mortality rate! Where do they obtain their proteins? The answer is simple: proteins are a part of virtually every natural food available to man. Every plant, every seed and every fruit contains some protein. It is virtually impossible not to obtain enough protein on any diet of *natural* foods, unless it is a starvation diet.

The long-held belief that meat proteins are superior to vegetable proteins has been disproved. Recent research has demonstrated that animal proteins in *any amounts* have a detrimental effect on health, and that vegetable proteins, formerly believed to be incomplete or inferior to animal proteins, *are actually biologically as good or better than animal proteins.*[3] Also, it has been

[3] Eimer, Karl, Professor (Klinik Schwenkenbacker), Zeitschrift für Ernahrung, July, 1933

scientifically demonstrated that good health can be sustained on a lesser amount of raw vegetable protein than cooked animal protein.[4] Potatoes are, for example, a good source of complete proteins which are biologically comparable to the proteins in eggs.[5]

2. *"YOU NEED MEAT PROTEIN FOR STRENGTH!"* Steak lovers like to think that meat gives them strength. The truth is exactly the opposite. Dr. Irving Fisher conducted endurance tests on vegetarians and meat-eaters which clearly showed the superior stamina of vegetarians. Then he lowered the content of protein in the diet of persons under the study and noticed that a 20 percent reduction in protein increased their endurance 33 percent.[6] Dr. R. Chittenden, of Yale University, made similar studies and demonstrated that muscle strength and endurance reaches its peak on about one-third of the usual protein intake. His explanation of this phenomenon is that animal protein metabolism results in a higher content of uric acid, urea and purines in the blood, and that these have a toxic effect on muscles and nerves.

3. *"YOU NEED LOTS OF PROTEINS EVERY DAY!"* This is another common fallacious notion. The fact that a person can live on a water or juice fast for months (one documented case of juice fasting is two hundred forty-nine days), without any proteins at all, proves that you don't have to *eat* proteins *every day,* although your body needs them each day. The proteins in your body are in a so-called dynamic state; they are constantly being decomposed and resynthesized. They are stored in blood plasma and used by the system as needed. During fasting, the inferior and diseased tissues are converted into useful

---

[4] DR. BIRCHER-BENNER'S WAY TO POSITIVE HEALTH AND VITALITY, Bircher-Benner Verlag, Zürich

[5] Schweigart, Prof. H. A. EIWEISS, FETTE, HERZINFARKT, Verlag H. H. Zauner, Munchen

[6] *Tidskrift för Hälsa,* Stockholm, November 1967

amino acids and stored in the liver or blood for immediate use.

So you don't need to *eat* proteins every day. Feel confident in taking short health-building fasts occasionally, or have a fruit-day now and then, without wondering "Where will I get my proteins?"

DO YOU NEED MEAT FOR SEXUAL VIRILITY?

In the previous chapter we have seen that animal meat was not considered by ancient nations an important virility-promoting food. In our "high-protein-cult" society, the belief persists that a fat steak equals a virile man. But men who depend on steak as the source of their sexual power may be cheating themselves and their wives. As Dr. George Belham, the author of THE VIRILITY DIET says:

> "The picture of a meat-eating male converting his food to muscle and brawn has as much basis as the claim that a roe-eating female is fertile . . . A large meat meal is more likely to make a man feel hot and sweaty than potent, especially in hot weather."[7]

Meat has a somewhat similar effect on sexual activity as some of the toxic aphrodisiacs described in the preceeding chapter. Those who do not eat meat regularly may feel a certain aphrodisiac effect after consuming a moderate meat meal. This is not so much due to meat's nutritional properties, as to the uric acid irritation on the mucous linings of the bladder, urethra and sexual apparatus.

Proteins are, of course, very essential nutrients for the peak of sexual power, make no mistake about that. Prolonged protein deficiency in the diet will definitely result in diminished interest in sex. But for these purposes,

---

[7] Belham, George, THE VIRILITY DIET, Dell Publishing Co., Inc., New York, 1968. Copyright (c) 1965 by George Belham

milk proteins have much to recommend them in preference to meat proteins. Milk is much more easily digested and assimilated and it does not have the adverse properties of meat. The occasional use of meat may be regarded as inducing sexual desire and potency, but prolonged and heavy consumption of animal meat will eventually have a detrimental effect on virility and may be a contributing cause to the growing loss of potency in the American male. The American male is the biggest meat eater in the world. According to statistics released recently by the National Livestock Meat Board, the average American male consumes 173 pounds of beef, pork, veal and lamb a year. This is nearly fifteen times the consumption of the Japanese male, who uses only 12.7 pounds of meat a year. In West Germany, the figure is 117 and in England 139 pounds.

Latin Americans, reputedly great lovers, eat only about one-third the amount of meat we eat. Does it not make you suspicious that the powerful high-protein propaganda, so lavishly sponsored by the meat packing industry in this country, is not giving you all the facts?

LIBIDO-DESTROYING ADDITIVES IN MEAT

In addition to the less desirable properties of meat for health generally and for virility in particular, mentioned so far, meat contains many toxic drugs used in animal feeding to speed the growth and fattening process. Residues of DDT and other chlorinated hydrocarbons, as well as such organophosphate pesticides as parathion, are found in almost all meat on the market today. Furthermore, meat is loaded with antibiotics and other drugs which are used in animal feed. Some of these drugs are left in meat when the animal is slaughtered, and they find their way to your dinner table.

In addition, most meats sold in America today, including

poultry and beef, have been fed rations containing *dietyl-stilbestrol,* a synthetic hormone. In Chapter 16 I have discussed in detail what this synthetic hormone can do for male virility and potency. If you eat lots of meat each day, you can be reasonably sure that you are receiving heavy daily doses of this hormone each day, since much of it remains in the carcass after the animal is killed. The authoritative drug manual, Merck Index, lists more than a dozen serious disorders which large doses of stilbestrol can cause in humans, including loss of libido in the male.

Perhaps a few generations back meat could have been considered a potent, energizing food. But if you look to meat today for masculine strength, it may have just the opposite effect. Stilbestrol-loaded meat may cause a further wilting of your virility.

VITAL POINTS IN THIS CHAPTER

1. High-protein requirement is a maxim in every American diet.
2. Notwithstanding the fact that virtually all authorities agree on this point, the importance of animal protein is overemphasized and the protein requirement tables are set too high.
3. Recent research shows that our actual protein need is lower than previously believed. The theory that animal proteins are more valuable than plant proteins, can no longer be scientifically justified.
4. The following beliefs:
    - You need meat for proteins
    - You need meat proteins for strength
    - You need lots of proteins every day
    - You need meat for masculine virility

are all fallacious, disproved by scientific research and/or empirical experience.

5. Animal proteins in today's chemicalized world are loaded with harmful drugs and chemical residues, and are not only hazardous to health generally but are also deleterious to masculinity and libido.

HOW TO PLAN A HIGH-VIRILITY DIET WITH A MINIMUM OF ANIMAL PROTEINS

1. Eliminate, or cut drastically, all meat from your diet. Remember: although men of every nation, race and continent have sought and used various substances to enhance and preserve their masculinity, meat has never been considered an important food for this purpose. Gland meats, such as liver and sex glands, enjoyed some popularity, but meat generally has been low on the list of desired virility foods.

2. If animal proteins are desired, fish, shellfish, and eggs are preferable to meat. Eggs are a time-tested virility food, especially egg yolks. Egg yolks are best eaten raw, but egg white should be cooked. It has been discovered that raw egg white contains a substance, *avidin,* that destroys biotin (one of the B-vitamins) in the intestinal tract. Cooking destroys the avidin.

3. Proteins *are* essential in a high-virility diet, but the best animal sources of protein for this purpose are milk and eggs. Milk has been rated highest in ancient virility diets as a protein source. This has been confirmed by modern investigations. The exceptional value of milk in this respect is, as explained by Dr. Leathem, of Rutgers University, due to the extraordinary high grade and complete nature of milk protein. *Casein,* milk protein, is the highest grade of protein known to man. It is more completely and easily digested and absorbed than any other form of protein. The highest grade protein is required by the pituitary gland in order to produce the hypophyseal hormone which stimu-

lates the activity of sex glands. Incidentally, milk proteins are just as valuable for the proper function of the female sexual system as for the male.

For the best biological value milk should be unpasteurized. Pasteurization destroys some vitamins along with possible pathogenic bacteria and makes some of the minerals and proteins biologically less valuable and less assimilable. Raw, unpasteurized milk is obtainable from better health food stores. Natural cheeses (not processed), such as Swiss, longhorn, Danish and cheddar, are also good sources of complete milk protein. One or two glasses of raw milk, a serving of cottage cheese and a couple of slices of good natural cheese on whole wheat bread will provide you with a generous amount of all the proteins you need for optimum health and virility. Add to this the proteins from your vegetables, potatoes, fruits and other foods, and you can stop worrying about getting enough proteins, even if you eliminate meat completely from your diet.

4. Other valuable sources of protein are: whole grains, raw nuts and seeds, especially almonds, peanuts, and sunflower seeds; sesame seeds; wheat germ; and brewer's or food yeast. Most of these items can be bought at health food stores. Use only whole-grain breads and cereals, which contain more proteins. Use wheat germ and brewer's yeast as food supplements. They are not only most excellent sources of proteins, but also of vitamins, minerals and trace elements.

5. Finally, almost everything you eat—provided it is not processed, refined or adulterated—contains valuable proteins. This is especially true of such vegetables as potatoes, yams and green leafy vegetables, which all contain *complete, top grade* proteins. Potatoes have acquired a wrong and damaging reputation as a pure starch, or carbohydrate food. Actually, potatoes are a good source of excellent proteins, which are comparable in biological value to egg proteins. Although the protein content per gram of potatoes is not

high, you usually eat a relatively larger portion of potatoes than of other protein foods. Therefore they can be a valuable source. In Germany, ten percent of daily protein need is obtained from potatoes. Potatoes are also rich in vitamin C and valuable minerals. But boil your potatoes with jackets on. Instant mashed potatoes are stripped of much of their nutritional value.

CHAPTER 9

HOW VITALIZING NUTRITION CAN BUILD A BASIS FOR HEALTHY AND HAPPY SEX LIFE

THE BASIC PREMISES upon which the message of this book is founded, are simple:

Number one: Nutrition is singularly the most important environmental factor affecting your health.

Number two: The health of your sexual and reproductive system is closely tied to and directly dependent on the general state of your health, particularly on the healthy functioning of your glandular system.

Thus, vital nutrition is a basis not only for buoyant health and long life, but also for a healthy and happy sex life.

These premises are not based on wishful thinking, but on established scientific facts. Today's doctors realize that they cannot talk about health or disease without talking about nutrition. Many other factors are involved, of course. But most medical scientists today agree that nothing can bring about as rapid and devastating a deterioration of health as faulty nutrition.

All agree that proper nutrition is imperative—*but what is proper nutrition?* The argument starts when we try to determine *what* constitutes a diet for optimum health.

FADS AND FACTS ABOUT NUTRITION

There are those who claim that "four basic food groups" will assure an adequate nutrition. Some believe that wheat and milk are harmful to health. There are vegetarians, raw food advocates, lacto-vegetarians and high-animal-protein cultists. There are many authorities who think that the prime health-destroying factors today are refined, devitalized, overprocessed foods, loaded with poisonous pesticide residues and toxic additives. Others assure us that nothing is wrong with our processed and chemicalized supermarket foods—they are just as nutritious as the so-called natural foods. And each one defends and supports his position with "mountains of scientific evidence," totally ignoring the other mountains of equally impressive evidence which prove his position erroneous.

So whom should the puzzled layman believe? Is it any wonder that he is ready to give up trying—and simply "eat what he likes?"

WHY UNIVERSAL DISAGREEMENT

Probably man started quarreling about food, what to eat and not to eat, as soon as he walked this earth. It is conceivable that Adam and Eve had more points of disagreement on food and nutrition than the renowned apple. It is equally reasonable to assume that man continued to argue about the value and the properties of foods throughout his long and colorful history; not only among the laymen, but among the enlightened and the learned as well.

The first great physician, Hippocrates, in his discourse on nutrition written almost five hundred years before Christ, says:

"If among those who had written on the subject

'which mode of living is the most health-promoting' was one who had grasped the matter in its whole width, I would be satisfied with his findings, learned from them and used them. Now, although many have written on the subject, none had a really full knowledge of what he was talking about—one had stressed one aspect, the other some other aspect, but none had hit the essence of the subject".[1]

Twenty-five hundred years later, Dr. Ralph Bircher of Zurich, Switzerland, wrote:

"I know of no branch of science more inclined to scholastic dogmatism and sentimental prejudice than nutrition. Health is a melancholy business."[2]

Dr. Bircher hits the nail on the head when he mentions "sentimental prejudice." Scientists and nutritionists are human. They are subjective in their judgments. We have to make provision for the human element even in the exact sciences. But medicine and nutrition are not exact sciences. Medicine is more an art than a science. When any given drug, vitamin, or food substance brings about a *different* reaction in every individual, you cannot talk about *exact science*.

Often, the results of "research" can hardly be considered dependable because the research is financed by interests which are looking for specific answers. The giant multi-billion-dollar food processing, chemical, and drug industries sponsor much of nutrition research in the United States, both in their own centers and in the form of grants to universities. "He who pays the piper, calls the tune." It would be naive to expect that such research would reveal the threat to American health today of overprocessed, devitalized foods, enormous drug consumption and a chemicalized, poisoned environment.

When scientific research is influenced by commercial

---

[1] CORPUS HIPPOCRATUM, quote translated by author

[2] DR. BIRCHER-BENNER'S WAY TO POSITIVE HEALTH AND VITALITY, Bircher-Benner Verlag, Zürich

interests the average layman is left wallowing in his own ignorance. One day he reads in the paper that tobacco causes cancer; the next day, a statement by another researcher that "there is no conclusive evidence . . ." One day he reads that fluoridation of water is harmful to his health —next day that it is beneficial. One scientist writes that processing of foods destroys vital nutrition and causes nutritional deficiency diseases—then another claims that modern processed foods are a boon. One authority will tell us that poisonous residues from pesticides in our foods are harming us in many ways—and a few days later we'll read the statement by another authority to the effect that the poison scare is a faddist's fantasy.

IS THERE ANY SOURCE AT ALL FOR RELIABLE, TRULY AUTHORITATIVE, SCIENTIFIC INFORMATION ON NUTRITION?

Fortunately, Yes.

Let me present this authority to you.

I.S.R.N.V.S.

The above initials stand for THE INTERNATIONAL SOCIETY FOR RESEARCH ON NUTRITION AND VITAL SUBSTANCES. It is an international organization, a voluntary union of professionals in medicine, nutrition, biochemistry and natural sciences from seventy-five countries. The Scientific Council of the Society includes four hundred prominent scientists from all over the world. One hundred twenty-one academic and other organizations dedicated to the promotion of health are incorporated members of the Society. About sixty-five percent of the members are medical doctors. The others represent allied branches of natural science. The Society is *absolutely independent* in its actions and research. *It is neither attached to nor supported by industry or by professional or economic interests or government.*

Dr. Albert Schweitzer was one of the original founders of this Society and its president until his death. The present president is a famous German scientist, Professor H. A. Schweigart. The list of member scientists includes a great number of Nobel Prize winners: the famous Vitamin C discoverer, Dr. A. Szent-Györgyi, the great Finnish scientist Dr. A. I. Virtanen, Professor Linus Pauling, Dr. J. Bernašek, from Czechoslavakia, Dr. B. W. Billow, Dr. R. M. Atwater and Dr. M. McCay from the United States, Dr. K. H. Karström from Sweden, etc., are on the Scientific Council of the Society. The recommendations made by the Society are the result of independent research by all these great men of science.

The Society's aim is to study the causes of diseases of civilization and to make a contribution through research to their reduction and prevention. The results of their research are made available to various governments and health organizations.

In today's labyrinth of conflicting ideas and opinions, the united report of this large and totally independent scientific forum is simply more to be trusted than the subjective opinions of self-appointed health experts—or the scattered research groups financed by special interests.

The following outline of vitalizing nutrition is based on the latest findings and recommendations of the International Society for Research on Nutrition and Vital Substances, as well as on available empirical evidence.

NATURAL FOODS SPELL OPTIMUM HEALTH AND FREEDOM FROM DISEASE

Natural foods are those grown without help of toxic chemicals or drugs and from which inherent nutritive values have not been removed by processing, heating or refining.

Here are a few examples:

Wheat, grown on fertile soils rich in humus, fertilized with manure and vegetable residues and consumed in the form of whole-grain products, is a *natural food*. Such natural whole-grain foods are rich in proteins, vitamins, minerals, enzymes. Such foods will not only supply you with potent nutrition, but also with vital enzymes which help your body to digest and utilize all nutritive factors. The wheat you eat in the form of white bread has little resemblance to natural wheat. First, it was grown on depleted soils with the help of chemical fertilizers, which means that its nutritive value to start with, was lower than that of wheat grown on fertile soil without chemical stimulation.

The protein content of today's wheat is twenty-five to thirty percent *lower* than it was a few generations back, before the chemical take-over of farming methods.

The nutritional value of wheat is further lowered by processing. Bran and wheat germ, which hold most of the vitamin B and E content, are removed in the milling process in order to make flour white and to increase its shelf life. The lifeless white powder is treated with bleaches and other chemicals which further lower its nutritional value. By the time the wheat reaches your table in the form of a white fluffy chemical concoction called bread, virtually none of the powerful nutritive values of wheat are left in it. In addition, it is loaded with various chemicals; pesticide residues, toxic preservatives, dough conditioners, softeners, mold inhibitors. After taking most of the natural vitamins and minerals and much of the protein out—over twenty nutrients in all—and adding only three synthetic B-vitamins and iron, they have gall to call this bread "enriched"! The chemical composition of wheat in white bread is altered and unbalanced. Vitamin E, important to the reproductive system of both men and women, is almost totally removed from white bread. Whole wheat is one of our best sources of vitamin E; but it would take two hundred slices of white bread to secure a proper daily requirement of this vital vitamin. The same goes for proteins, minerals, and B-vitamins. Yet, there are "authorities" who tell you that no nutritional difference exists between whole-grain bread and fortified white bread.

Eggs are another case in point. Natural eggs, laid by hens living in a natural outdoor environment, enjoying fresh air, sunshine—and, don't forget, a rooster!—and eating their natural food in the form of insects, worms, grass and seeds (grains), are natural eggs, full of nutritive value. But today's eggs, produced in egg "factories" by chicks who never see the sun or green grass, *or a rooster,* and who are fed only synthetic medicated mash, are not natural eggs. Such eggs are sterile, i.e. they will not produce chickens, their chemical composition is altered and unbalanced, and their vitamin content is lower. Look at the difference in the color of the yolks! The total nutritional value of such eggs is much lower than that of natural eggs.

Natural foods, grown under natural conditions, unprocessed and unrefined, contain more proteins, more vitamins, and particularly more vital enzymes, than denatured foods.

One more extremely important reason exists for eating natural foods. Although the science of nutrition has made a terrific leap forward in the past few decades, our knowledge of vital substances in foods is incomplete. New vitamins and other substances are discovered frequently. We may reasonably assume that in the future many new nutritive elements will be found in natural foods. Scientists who tried to feed test animals a synthetic diet which contained *all the nutritive substances known to science* have found that the animals could live in seemingly good health for a while. But after the second or third generation their health started to deteriorate and specifically their reproductive capacity was weakened. Finally they totally lost their power to reproduce and the whole strain eventually died.[3] These scientific experiments show that natural foods contain vital substances yet unknown to science. When you eat natural foods you will obtain not only all the known nutritive factors, but also have the benefit of the undiscovered substances as well.

Milk and milk products which, as we pointed out in the previous chapter, are important for your health and for your virility, should also come from healthy animals which were fed natural, organically-grown fodder and not from the artificial diet of hormones, antibiotics and poisonous chemical residues which find their way through the milk into your system.

More than ninety per cent of all foods we eat today have been tampered with in one way or another. Many of the important nutrients present in natural whole foods have been removed or destroyed. White sugar, white bread, processed cereals, canned foods and processed oils are devitalized and denatured. We are using more and more so-called "convenience" foods in preference to natural foods. The consumption of fresh fruits and vegetables per capita in the United States has declined one third since 1930, according to the U.S. Department of Agriculture. At the same time we consume twenty-five billion dollars worth of processed cereals, baked goods, soft drinks, macaroni, confectionary and other nutrition-less empty calories, which can produce nothing but disease and diminished virility.

That your health and your vitality are in direct relationship to the *naturalness* of the foods you eat is a

---

[3] Bernašek, J. M.D. THE BANKRUPTCY OF SYNTHETIC FOODS, *Tidskrift för Hälsa,* December, 1964

solid scientific fact. Dr. Weston A. Price, D.D.S., made an extensive study of diet habits as related to the health of practically every people in the world. He has found that where people lived on natural, unprocessed, fresh foods, grown in their own environment, they had no tooth decay or disease. They were strong, virile and happy. They enjoyed long lives. Conversely, Dr. Price found that where people ate denatured, cooked, processed foods, especially white sugar and white flour, they were subject to tooth decay and various diseases peculiar to civilized man.

The Hunza Kingdom in India is a good example of the value of natural foods. Isolated by inaccessible mountains, Hunzakuts have no way of obtaining white sugar, white flour, or canned or processed foods. Their diet consists of unadulterated grains, vegetables, fruits and animal foods produced without chemicals. Hunzakuts are called "the healthiest people in the world." The British physician, Dr. R. McCarrison, lived among them for eleven years trying to find traces of diseases common to civilized man. He concluded that "they know no sickness." They live to be ninety or one hundred and are virile, strong and active long after they pass the proverbial three score and ten. Hunza men are known to have fathered children after the age of one hundred.

LIVING FOODS FOR PEAK OF HEALTH AND VITALITY

Man seems to use inventiveness and imagination in devising ever newer ways of ruining his food. The first major step in this direction, which started man's slow degeneration to the present inferno of ill health, was the discovery of *cooking*.

"Man is the only creature upon this earth who spoils his food before he eats it," said Dr. Robert Bell. Man has devised countless ways to "spoil" his food: by processing, refining, adding toxic preservatives and other chemicals, freezing, canning and so forth. His latest discovery is irradiation. It is too early to say what exactly this irradiation with atomic rays will do to the life-sustaining power of food. It kills the germinating capacity in foods—will it do the same to the people who eat such foods? There is growing concern among responsible scientists that man's reproductive powers are already threatened by all the chemicals in his food and environment. Physiologically speaking, you are what you eat—and devitalized foods create devitalized people.

But perhaps the worst—although the least suspected—way to devitalize food and lower its nutritional value, that man has ever devised, was also the first—cooking. Cooking (boiling, frying, baking) lowers the nutritional value of food in many ways:

- Cooking destroys *all* enzymes.
- Cooking destroys many nutrients, especially vitamins C and B, which are vulnerable to heat.
- Cooking in water soaks minerals and water-soluble vitamins out of the food, which are then usually thrown away with the cooking water.
- Cooking changes the biochemical structure of proteins and fats and makes them more difficult to be digested and assimilated.

ENZYMES—THE MIRACLE LIFE-FORCE

Enzymes are vital catalysts, absolutely essential for your health. Without enzymes your body cannot properly digest and assimilate nourishment. Although a certain amount of enzymes are manufactured within your body, food enzymes are needed for effective digestion. Enzymes are also needed for the healthy function of practically all organs of your body. Without them, you would starve to death even if you ate the most nutritious foods in the world, because your body would not be able to utilize the nutrients you gave it. As important as vitamins, minerals and proteins are, without enzymes they are powerless. Enzymes transform food substances into living cells and into your vital organs and glands. Your physical and mental energy, your brain capacity, your resistance to disease and stress, your sexual power—all depend on the magic work of enzymes.

The following dramatic story tells how the powerful effect of enzymes was discovered and how a young girl's life was saved.

A Swiss physician had a young patient who was dying of starvation. Her stomach could digest nothing she ate. The doctor tried everything, from medication to every imaginable diet, to no avail. Morning tests showed that all the food she had eaten the evening before remained completely undigested in her stomach. The girl was emaciated and not expected to live more than a few days.

The disheartened doctor confided his concern to an amateur student of ancient scripts. The doctor's friend remembered that in the writings of Pythagoras, a diet of raw fruits with raw goat's milk and natural honey was used in cases of indigestion. The friend suggested that the doctor try this old prescription.

The doctor was horrified. Give a dying patient, who could not digest even finely mashed and well-cooked foods, a diet of raw fruit? This was contrary to all the practices and all elementary dietetic rules he had learned in medical school. But his patient was dying and he had nothing else to try. He discussed the idea with the patient, who agreed to the experiment and assumed responsibility for the trial.

The raw food dish was prepared and fed to the patient. The doctor expected the worst. But to his surprise, the next morning the patient felt better. Tests showed that for the first time her food was completely digested in her stomach.

The same foods, cooked, had been totally undigested; in raw form, they seemed to digest easily. The doctor continued feeding his patient raw food. Eventually her health was completely restored. Her life had been saved by a twenty-five-hundred-year-old raw food recipe.

This happened in 1895. The doctor's name was Max Bircher-Benner. He later became world-famous by restoring thousands of patients' health in his sanatorium in Zurich, primarily through therapies based on the "life-force" factor in raw foods. Enzymes had not even been discovered at that time. Although Dr. Bircher-Benner could not pinpoint the vital curative force he discovered, this fact did not prevent him from using the discovery for the benefit of thousands of sick people.

Now we know that this life force was *enzymes*. The atrophied digestive system of the young girl was not capable of utilizing food because all her food was well-cooked and totally lacking in essential enzymes. When she ate raw foods, she could digest and utilize the nutrients from them because raw foods contain all the enzymes needed for their own digestion. Raw, living foods are able to digest themselves.

ENZYMES AND VIRILITY

If you recall from the list of aphrodisiac foods used by ancients, which we discussed in Chapter 7, goat's milk, honey, and apples were high on the list of such foods. The reason for this is not difficult to understand. Raw milk proteins are the most easily digested and utilized of all proteins known to man. Goat's milk is even better in this respect than cow's milk, because it is naturally homogenized. Honey is, of course, one of the best known aphrodisiac and rejuvenating foods, its value being confirmed by modern research. Apples have the same traditional reputation. These three foods are wonder-health-foods and powerful storehouses of enzymes.

Primitive man lived on raw foods—nuts, honey, seeds and raw milk—and enjoyed excellent health. With the discovery of cooking and other ways of processing and preserving foods, the amount of raw food in man's diet has gradually diminished. At the same time diseases are on the increase. Although many infectious diseases of the past have been conquered, mainly because of improved sanitation and better hygiene, the degenerative diseases are on the increase at an alarming speed. Almost half the population of the United States is chronically ill. Man's fertility and sexual health are on the decline too. We have seen a tremendous increase in sterile marriages, miscarriages, malformed babies and other reproductive disorders. Man's bad living habits, particularly his devitalized foods, are to a large degree to blame for his deteriorating health.

Enzymes are magic workers for your health. They increase your resistance to disease. They speed the healing process when you are sick. They can keep you young and virile. Their chemical action on the glandular functions determines the amount of hormones produced and released by your glands.

Only living foods, in a natural, unprocessed state, contain all the enzymes needed for the functions of your body. Enzymes are totally destroyed in cooking, and largely destroyed by various methods of processing.

Therefore, to benefit from the powerful effect of enzymes on your health and virility, eat as many raw foods as possible. All fruits and vegetables should be eaten raw. Nuts, milk, honey and seeds, such as sunflower seeds, should be eaten raw, not pasteurized, heated, or toasted. Practically all foods in their raw state are easier to digest than cooked foods.

If you are now eating largely "dead" foods, start the transition to living foods gradually, to give your digestive system time to rebuild itself and adapt to the new diet. Gradually add more and more raw foods to your diet until you arrive at a program where at least two-thirds of all your food is eaten raw. Not only are raw foods better for you, they also taste better. Egg yolks should be eaten raw. Fish can be eaten raw too; the Japanese have many ways of preparing raw fish. Enzymes in meat can also be partly preserved by undercooking rather than overcooking—raw steaks are certainly more acceptable from a nutritional standpoint than well done ones—if you still want meat after reading the previous chapter. Most grains can be sprouted and eaten raw—another potent health and virility food. Obtain a brochure from your favorite health food store on how to sprout seeds and grains. Start using these sprouts in your daily diet. You may be surprised at the powerful revitalizing effect they have on your body.

Only living foods can give you maximum vitality.

POISONS IN FOOD CAN HARM YOUR HEALTH AND LOWER YOUR VIRILITY

In the opinion of many doctors, poisons in food and environment present the greatest modern threat to health. We are subjected to never-ending toxic assault from every direction. It is almost impossible to obtain food free from poisonous residue. Fruits and vegetables contain residues of harmful insecticides, waxes and artificial colorings; milk and butter contain heavy doses of DDT; meat and poultry contain residues of antibiotics, DDT, synthetic hormones and other drugs used to speed the animals' growth and fattening process. Processed meats, bread, cereals, and canned foods and drinks contain a great number of preservatives, artificial coloring and flavorings and other harmful substances. Nearly one thousand chemicals are used today in the food processing industry. Many have never been tested for toxicity.

Are all these poisons in our food and our environment

really harming our health, or is this just alarmist talk? As much as we would like to believe otherwise, *these poisons are more harmful than we can even imagine*. There is a growing concern among world scientists that we are slowly committing mass suicide with all these poisons. The multi-billion-dollar food-processing industry, blinded by greed and looking for more profits, keeps adding more and more poisonous chemicals to our food and drink. Our soil, our rivers, our drinking water and our air are growing more toxic with every passing year. Warnings are voiced by many responsible scientists and organizations, including the International Society for Research on Nutrition and Vital Substances, that *it is later than we think* and that unless we stop further poisoning of our food and our planet, we will have to face a gradual extinction of all life. These warnings go unnoticed. Many concerned scientists think that we have already reached the point of no return.

Propaganda tries to convince us that we are the best fed and the healthiest nation in the world. Those who question the chemicals used in food processing are labeled "nutritional quacks" and "alarmists." People are mass-hypnotized by clever advertising into buying worthless, nutrition-less so-called foods. Realizing that not all adults are that easily fooled, vendors appeal in their commercials to the youngsters and command them "go and tell your mom" to buy their product. This is so skillfully done that many mothers and wives today are conscientiously feeding their families nutritionally worthless diets.

POISONS AND SEXUAL HEALTH

What effect do all these poisons in man's food and environment have on his sexual health?

Animal studies have demonstrated that insecticides can cause sterility. Insecticides cause hormonal imbalance in the system and can lead to infertility.[4] It also has been demonstrated that stilbestrol can cause loss of masculinity and diminished virility (see Chapter 16).

One of the most common poisons in our food, air, and water is lead, which comes chiefly from the lead-containing gasolines used in automobiles. Lead is a lethal poison and can harm you in many ways. It interferes with the fertility of both men and women. Severe lead poisoning may cause miscarriage, premature births, stillbirths and even total sterility. Chronic lead poisoning can cause sexual impotence in men.[5]

The reproductive systems of both men and women are adversely affected by the polluted environment. Dr. James Crow, the Chairman of the National Institute of Health's Genetics Study Section, said there are strong indications that some of the chemicals in man's environment—food, air, water—can cause damage to our genes and chromosomes. "There is no reason to think that we are exempt," said Dr. Crow. Captan, a widely used agricultural fungicide —which many home gardeners spray on roses—was recently suspected of being mutagenic, or mutation-causing. Many of our nation's geneticists are alarmed by the potential mutagenic chemicals which enter our environment. A river of chemicals surrounds all of us, possibly causing damage to our genes and, therefore, to our unborn babies.

Smog, a growing menace, is directly singled out as a possible cause of genetic damage. Dr. A. J. Haagen-Smit, professor of biology at the California Institute of Technology, says recent laboratory studies show that oxides of nitrogen—carbon monoxide and other toxic gases from automobiles—cause mutations. A "distinct possibility" exists that city smog may affect people's genes and thus

---

[4] Farris, Edmond J., M.D., *Prevention,* January 1969

[5] Willy, A., M.D., et al., THE ILLUSTRATED ENCYCLOPEDIA OF SEX, Cadillac Publishing Co., N.Y., 1965

change the inherited characteristics of our descendents.

Birth defects are a fast-growing problem in the United States. At present, seven percent of all children born have some form of defect or abnormality.[6] Some scientists believe that the drugs and chemicals we use are involved in teratogenicity—the birth of deformed babies. Radiation is also named among possible causes of birth defects. Recently the FDA started a hurried investigation when some of our most commonly used artificial sweeteners were suddenly suspected of causing genetic damage. And of course, we all know the tragedy of thalidomide.

All in all, it is obvious that the never-ending stream of chemicals, dangerous drugs and poisons in our food, air, and water can have nothing but detrimental effects on our health and consequently on the health of our reproductive system.

FIVE BASIC RULES OF NUTRITION FOR OPTIMUM HEALTH AND A HEALTHY AND HAPPY SEX LIFE

1. *Number one* rule of optimum nutrition is the *naturalness* of your food. Only whole, unrefined, unadulterated foods can produce optimum health. Food grown in depleted soils with the help of chemicals; refined and processed foods from which most of the natural nutritive factors have been removed or destroyed; meat, eggs, and milk from animals who are fed synthetic chemicalized food and hormones—these are not natural foods. They are biologically and nutritionally inferior to natural foods, have lower nutritional value and can produce nothing but a lower state of health.

Avoid processed cereals, white sugar and white flour

---

[6] Nishimura, Hideo, M.D., CHEMISTRY AND PREVENTION OF CONGENITAL ANOMALIES, Charles C. Thomas, Publisher, 1964

in every form, hydrogenated fats, processed and hormone-grown meats, pasteurized or imitation milk. Better health food stores usually carry organically grown produce, fruits and whole-grain products grown without chemicals. They also sell raw, unpasteurized milk and cheese, unprocessed cold-pressed vegetable oils and other natural products. Only whole, unrefined foods contain all the vitamins, minerals, proteins and other vital substances which you need for optimum health and peak sexual virility.

2. *Number two* rule of vitalizing nutrition for optimum health is that you should eat *living foods*. Cooking alters the biochemical structure of food and tends to make it less digestible and assimilable. Cooking also destroys enzymes.

Eat most of your food raw. If cooking is required, cook as little as possible at low heat to preserve enzymes and other nutrients. Potatoes, yams, squash and such, should be baked or cooked in very little water with skins on. Nuts, seeds and grains should be eaten raw if possible. Sprouted grains are storehouses of enzymes and vitamins. Not less than a half, still better two-thirds, of all you eat should be raw, if you want to attain a peak of health and vitality.

3. *Number three* rule of wholesome nutrition in today's poisoned world is that your food should be as *poison-free* as possible. Poisons in your food, water and air are *definitely* harming your health and the health of your reproductive system.

How are you to avoid these poisons which threaten your health from every direction? I wish I could give you a satisfactory answer, but I can't. Should you move to a distant, isolated Pacific Island and enjoy pure air and natural, unprocessed, poison-free native foods? Even this would not solve the problem, because our "great chemical progress" has already succeeded in poisoning this planet so thoroughly that fish, birds, and animals in the most distant parts of the globe, even in Arctic and Antarctic regions, have been found to contain traces of DDT in their tissues. Then what can we do—just resign and witness the slow but inevitable mass-suicide-through-chemistry process? Regretfully, there is not much we can do . . . but we must try. Here are some things we can do to protect ourselves from the ever-present poisons:

- If at all possible, move to an area which is not affected by *smog*.
- Make every effort to obtain *organically-grown* fruits and vegetables. They are usually sold in health food stores; or you may be able to locate an organic farm and buy directly.

  If at all possible, have your own backyard garden and grow your own poison-free vegetables (provided you do not live close to heavy traffic, in which case even your backyard vegetables will be loaded with lead).
- If you have to depend on your supermarket for vegetables and fruits, wash them carefully to remove the traces of toxic chemicals. In some European sanatoriums, a hydrochloric solution is used to remove traces of insecticide. This is how they do it:

  One percent hydrochloric solution is made by mixing one ounce of pure hydrochloric acid from the drug store with three quarts of water. Use only a glass, enamel or earthenware utensil. Wash fruits and vegetables well, place them in the solution for five minutes, rinse thoroughly and brush them well. The solution can be reused for about a week.

4. HIGH-NATURAL-CARBOHYDRATE — LOW-ANIMAL-PROTEIN DIET is the diet most conducive to optimum health and vitality. As you have seen in Chapter 8, proteins are essential in optimum-health-and-virility diet. But the

importance of animal meat in a diet is definitely over-emphasized by most American authorities. Recent research shows that our actual protein needs are lower than previously estimated. The proteins from vegetable and milk are as valuable as meat proteins, without meat's adverse effects on health. In addition, today's meat contains many harmful drugs, chemicals and hormones, which are deleterious factors on the health and sexual virility.

The Scientific Council of the International Society for Research on Nutrition and Vital Substances, after a seven-year study of all available scientific data on nutrition, recommends the following dietary program:

> "A complete well-balanced diet with the greatest potential of building optimal health and preventing diseases of old age, should have the following characteristics:
>
> - Natural, whole, unadulterated foods, free from harmful additives;
> - An adequate supply of vital substances (vitamins, proteins, minerals, enzymes, essential fatty acids, trace elements, etc.)
> - A moderate supply of calorie and energy-producing foods of carbohydrate category.
> - A lacto-veggtarian diet of fresh foods (a diet based on whole grain products, vegetables, fruits, seeds and nuts, and milk and milk products).
>
> Raw, unprocessed milk is especially recommended as a protein, vitamin, and mineral-rich food.
>
> Meat, fish, and eggs can supplement this diet, but their daily use is not necessary.
>
> This basic diet should be enriched by such natural, unprocessed and untreated foods as fruit juices, nuts, flaxseed, whole-grain cereals, soured milk, yogurt, kefir, all available fresh berries and fruits, honey, cold-pressed vegetable oils and edible yeast (brewer's yeast).

The importance of honey in the diet of older people is especially emphasized."

So here we have it, from the most authoritative scientific source! The macrobiotic diet with the greatest potential for health and vitality: a *high-natural-carbohydrate —low-animal protein diet.*

A special note on meat: although meat is considered a virility food by many Americans, this is more a reflection of the general high-protein myth, than a scientifically supported fact. Heavy meat consumption is definitely detrimental to health and, consequently, detrimental to sexual health. An occasional meat meal may have a certain stimulating effect but continued overindulgence in meat will eventually lead to a diminished libido, if for no other reason than because of the libido-destroying stilbestrol most meat contains today. The best proteins for sexual health are those from milk, cheese, eggs, seafood, and vegetables.

5. *Finally*, it's not *what you eat*, but *what you assimilate* that counts! You may eat the most nourishing food in the world but if your digestive system is not able to utilize this food, it won't do you any good. Food must be broken down to small molecules which can be assimilated by the bloodstream and transformed into living cells by the action of enzymes. Faulty digestion and poor assimilation of food can be brought about in the following ways:

- *Overeating.* "A full belly is the mother of all evil," said Benjamin Franklin. Russian statistics show that one common characteristic of people who lived one hundred years or more and enjoyed good health and vitality, is that throughout their lives they were moderate eaters. Fat people are poor lovers. Obesity not only decreases life expectancy, but also decreases sexual potency. Dr. C.M. McCay, of Cornell University, has shown in extensive experiments that overeating is the major cause of premature aging.
- *Hurried eating.* Slow eating and good mastication

are essential for good digestion and assimilation of food. Good chewing starts the digestion of food in your mouth, increases its assimilation in the intestinal tract and makes you feel satisfied with a lesser amount of food.

- *Lack of relaxation after eating.* You should always eat in a relaxed atmosphere and enjoy what you are eating. Only the food you have enjoyed can do you any good. But it is also important that you take a short rest after each meal. The digestion of the food requires a great amount of blood. This blood is temporarily withdrawn from your brain, your muscles, your sexual apparatus . . . To plunge into heavy mental or physical work—or sexual activity—right after a big meal is a health-destroying practice. It will lead to poor digestion and assimilation, putrefaction in the intestinal tract and possible gastric disorders.

INSTANT OR LONG-TERM VIRILITY

A diet built on the principles outlined here will result in better health and greater resistance to disease and stress. It will also increase your vitality, give you more energy and pep, strengthen your physical and mental powers. Since sexual vitality is closely tied to your general health, it is self-evident that improved health may also result in improved sexual performance.

This program is, however, not aimed at a quick, instant stimulus to your amatory powers. It is a long-term virility program, aimed at building and strengthening your general health and preventing premature aging—physically, mentally and sexually. This program will bring you optimum health. And optimum health is your best guarantee for a robust and happy sex life as long as you live.

BRIEF SUMMARY OF THIS CHAPTER

1. Nutrition is the most important environmental factor affecting your health.

2. The health of your sexual and reproductive system is closely tied to the general state of your health and, consequently, your nutrition.

3. What is proper nutrition? Which foods are health-promoting and which are not? The most dependable, authoritative source of scientific information on matters of nutrition and health.

4. A five-point program of vitalizing nutrition for optimum health and a happy sex life, based on recommendations by The International Society for Research on Nutrition and Vital Substances.

CHAPTER 10

HOW VITAMINS, MINERALS, AND TRACE ELEMENTS AFFECT YOUR SEX LIFE

THE SCIENCE OF nutrition is relatively new. Although man has throughout history recognized the paramount value of good nutrition, he has lacked the exact knowledge as to which factors in foods make them beneficial. He has been guided by purely empirical evidence based on experience. In 2500 B.C., Hippocrates, the Father of Medicine, said: "Our food must be our medicine—our medicine must be our food."

The discovery of vitamins with their role in health or disease, was one of the greatest scientific achievements of all time. Millions of people are living today or feeling well, who would have been either dead or hopelessly ill, were it not for vitamin and mineral therapies.

Vitamins and minerals are absolutely essential for your health. Without them you would perish. They constitute a vital part of nutrition. Even minor vitamin deficiencies in the diet may cause serious deficiency diseases and a generally lowered condition of health.

Vitamins and enzymes are catalysts which influence and trigger all the vital processes in your body including sexual activity. Minerals are equally important. They are needed for all important metabolic processes in your body. The proper chemical balance in your tissues is imperative for your health—minerals are responsible for maintaining this balance. A disordered biochemical balance in the system is considered by many researchers to be the prime cause of most disease.

VITAMINS AND MINERALS FOR SEXUAL POWER

Directly and indirectly, vitamins and minerals are involved in your sexual health. Foods have a profound effect on your sexual activity largely because of their vitamin and mineral content. Here are a few examples:

- Vitamin A is needed for maintaining testicular tissue in a healthy state.[1] It is also needed for healthy mucous membranes in the reproductive organs.
- Several of the B-vitamins are needed before sex hormones can be produced.[2]
- Vitamin E is needed for normal sex hormone production, for a healthy condition of the ovaries and testes, and for prevention of miscarriage. A deficiency of vitamin E can cause male and female sterility. Vitamin E also protects sex hormones from destruction by oxidation.[3]
- Phosphorous is needed for the normal healthy function of the brain, nerves and the sexual nerve centers.

[1] Walton, A. H., APHRODISIACS FROM LEGEND TO PRESCRIPTION, Associated Booksellers, Bridgeport, Conn. 06606

[2] Davis, Adelle, LET'S GET WELL, Harcourt, Brace & World, Inc., N.Y., 1965

[3] Beckman, R., Costa, A., et al., *International Congress on Vitamin E.*, 1955

- Zinc, a trace element, is vital to the health of the prostate gland. A deficiency of zinc in the diet can cause malfunction of the prostate, retarded genital development and poor sexual performance.

Of course, the action of most vitamins, minerals and trace elements on sexual activity is indirect, through their effect on the glandular activity and on the body functions generally. Vitamin E, for example, in addition to its direct effect on sexual glands, has a profound effect on sexual activity through its action on the anterior lobe of the pituitary, which has control over sexual activity. Another example of indirect effect is the stimulating effect of vitamins E and C on the thyroid gland. Thyroid hormones give your body much of its libido. An underactive thyroid gland can make a young man lose his interest in sex. Thus, vitamin and mineral deficiency can cause diminished endocrine hormone production and resultant diminished libido.

HOW PREVALENT ARE VITAMIN DEFICIENCIES?

Although scurvy and pellagra, the most pronounced vitamin deficiency diseases, are relatively rare in the United States, sub-clinical vitamin and mineral deficiencies are wide-spread. According to a 1968 report by the U.S. Department of Agriculture, one in every five families has a nutritionally poor diet. Vitamin deficiencies are particularly prevalent among young people of high school and college age.

In a country with the most abundant food supply in the world, why are so many malnourished? The answer is ignorance. "People just don't know what kind of foods are necessary for good health and vigor," said Assistant Secretary of Agriculture, George L. Mehren.

With this introduction, let us now look at the various vitamins, minerals and trace elements and see what relation they have to our health.

VITAMIN A

Vitamin A from vegetable foods is usually first found in the form of carotene, which is converted in the body into vitamin A. The animal foods, eggs and milk contain the actual vitamin.

Vitamin A is one of our most important vitamins and it is involved in many vital body processes. Here are a few examples:

- It promotes growth in the child.
- It is extremely important for your eyes; it prevents eye diseases and counteracts night blindness.
- It is a "membrane conditioner"—it keeps mucous linings of your body, including the mucous linings of sexual and reproductive organs, in good condition.
- It helps to maintain testicular tissue in a healthy state.
- It is an anti-infection vitamin, it protects you against colds, flu and other infections.
- It aids in the secretion of gastric juices and in the digestion of proteins.
- It plays a vital part in nourishing your skin and hair.
- It helps to prevent premature aging and increases life expectancy, as demonstrated by Dr. H.C. Sherman of Columbia University. Vitamin A regulates the stability of tissue in cell walls, as reported by another Columbia University scientist, Dr. Oswald A. Roels. Cell membranes break down when there is a lack of vitamin A.

A deficiency of vitamin A in the diet can result in eye inflammations, frequent colds and other acute infections, retarded growth in children, degenerative changes in mucous membranes, rough dry skin and such skin disorders as acne, pimples, boils and psoriasis. Doctors use large daily doses of vitamin A to treat skin disorders, eye conditions, and infections—50,000 to 100,000 I.U. (International Units) or even higher. The official recommended daily dietary allowance is 5,000 units.

The best natural sources of vitamin A are carrots, green leafy vegetables (such as turnip greens and spinach) sweet potatoes, kale, melon, squash, tomatoes, eggs, butter, peaches, apricots and—last but not least—fish liver oils, the richest source of all.

HOW TO FORTIFY YOUR DIET WITH VITAMIN A

1. Eat fresh carrots, tomatoes and green leafy vegetables each day.
2. Drink freshly made carrot juice.
3. Take cod liver oil capsules as a food supplement (obtainable at all health food stores or drug stores). Up to 25,000 units a day is a safe dosage. Vitamin A in capsule form is easy to take and has no unpleasant fishy taste.

VITAMIN B-COMPLEX

There are many vitamins with diversified properties which belong to the B-family of vitamins, called B-complex. The best understood B-vitamins are thiamine, riboflavin, niacin, pyridoxine, biotin, pantothenic acid, B_{12} B_{15}, para-aminobenzoic acid, folic acid, choline and inositol.

THIAMINE (B_1) is called the age-fighting vitamin. It protects the heart muscle, it stimulates the brain action and is indispensible for the health of the entire nervous system. A gross deficiency of thiamine causes beriberi. Thiamine is needed for effective digestion of carbohydrates. Natural carbohydrate foods, therefore, are always accompanied by thiamine, vitamin B_1. When you eat refined carbohydrates, such as white sugar and white bread, your body must use its own storage supplies of thiamine in order to digest the carbohydrates properly. This will eventually lead to thiamine deficiency. A chronic lack of thiamine in the diet may cause insomnia, constipation, digestive disorders, loss of weight and appetite and muscle weakness.

The minimum daily requirement of thiamine is 1.2 milligrams.

RIBOFLAVIN (B_2) affects the health of your skin, nails and hair. One of the most common symptoms of a serious deficiency of B_2 in the diet are cracks on the lips and a sore, burning tongue. Dull hair, premature wrinkles on face and arms, and split fingernails are other typical symptoms of riboflavin deficiency.

The minimum daily requirement is 1.7 milligrams.

NIACIN (nicotinic acid) is best known as the anti-pellagra vitamin. It may also prevent migraine headaches. Niacin dilates small blood capillaries and increases the flow of blood to the peripheral capillary system. It is prescribed by doctors in cases of cold feet and hands.

The recommended daily requirement is 15 milligrams.

PYRIDOXINE (B_6) is involved in protein metabolism, in the production of antibodies which protect from bacterial invasion, in the function of the nervous system and is important for normal reproductive processes. A deficiency of B_6 may lead to anemia, nervous disorders and insomnia.

The recommended daily need is 1.5 milligrams.

BIOTIN (vitamin H) has recently been found to relate to hair growth. Biotin is involved in the metabolism of proteins and fats. Biotin deficiency can cause fat dandruff which contributes to hair loss, seborrhea, lack of appetite, eczema, fatigue, confusion, irritability and mental depression. A certain amount of biotin is produced in the intestines.

The daily requirement is 150 to 300 micrograms.

PANTOTHENIC ACID is known as the anti-gray vitamin. Its stabilizing action on the adrenal glands may prevent graying of the hair. Pantothenic acid, one of the most versatile B-vitamins, is involved in almost all vital body processes. It increases cortisone production, protects you in times of stress, increases your vitality, wards off infections and speeds recovery from ill health. Deficiency of pantothenic acid can cause chronic fatigue, increased tendency to infection, loss of hair, mental depressions and irritability.

The daily requirement is 8 to 10 milligrams.

VITAMIN B_{12} is essential for the production of red blood cells. The deficiency of vitamin B_{12} can cause anemia, irregular menstruation and vaginal discharge.

VITAMIN B_{15} (pangamic acid) helps to regulate fat metabolism, heightens oxygen assimilation in the tissues, stimulates the glandular and nervous systems and is helpful in the treatment of heart disease. Recently, Russian doctors used B_{15} successfully to treat hypoxia, or oxygen deficiency in tissues. They have found that vitamin B_{15} increased the body's tolerance to lowered oxygen supply. This is of special importance in the United States because of our nation-wide air pollution problem. Carbon monoxide induces hypoxia by preventing oxygen from being absorbed by the lungs. Vitamin B_{15} can help us to protect ourselves from slow carbon monoxide poisoning.

PARAAMINOBENZOIC ACID (PABA) has been used experimentally in attempts to restore natural color to grey hair, soothe the pain of burns, treat stubborn cases of eczemas and sunburns. Indications are that PABA can prevent old-age skin changes.

FOLIC ACID (B_9), like vitamin B_{12}, is involved in the blood-building process and also in new cell production. Folic acid is important for the health of the skin. A deficiency of folic acid can cause serious skin disorders and loss of hair. When folic acid is returned to the diet, the hair begins to grow normally.

CHOLINE and *INOSITOL* are two B-vitamins that co-operate in preventing hardening of the arteries and protecting the kidneys and liver. They are involved in fat metabolism and promote the normal distribution of fat throughout the body. Choline is necessary for the manufacture of a substance in the blood called phospholipid. Inositol is also vital for hair growth.

The recommendation for minimum daily need for inositol varies between 1 and 3 grams, but the exact requirement for choline has not been established. It is, however, believed that a deficiency of choline in America is common, and that our daily intake of choline is considerably less than the actual requirement.

THE BEST NATURAL SOURCES OF VITAMIN B-COMPLEX

Foods rich in B-vitamins are:

- All whole-grain products, especially whole-wheat bread and cereals.
- Wheat germ and wheat bran.
- Seeds, nuts, beans and peas. Sunflower seeds, pumpkin seeds, raw peanuts, almonds and soybeans are good sources of B-vitamins in addition to being excellent protein foods.
- Beef and calf liver (including B_{12}).
- Milk and cheese (including B_{12}).
- Vegetables and fruits, such as kale, turnip greens, cabbage, grapefruit, cauliflower, watermelon and spinach.
- Brewer's yeast—the richest natural source of B-complex vitamins.

HOW TO FORTIFY YOUR DIET WITH B-VITAMINS

1. Use only whole grain bread and cereals. Use plenty of beans, peas, and such foods as sunflower seeds and sesame seeds (in the form of Halvah, see Chapter 11 for recipe and instructions).
2. Add fresh raw wheat germ to your breads or sprinkle a tablespoon of it over your salads and cereals.
3. Take one or two tablespoons of brewer's yeast (or equivalent in tablets) each day. Brewer's yeast tablets or powder are sold in every health food or drug store.
4. Take two teaspoons of lecithin each day for choline and inositol.
5. Eat milk and cheese regularly.
6. If you eat meat—have liver once a week.

VITAMIN C

The most important function of vitamin C is keeping the collagen—the intercellular cement—in a healthy condition. Collagen is the substance which keeps all your tissues together—in bones, teeth, muscles, skin, blood vessels and vital organs. A deficiency of vitamin C can cause the deterioration of the collagen and consequently the breakdown of tensile strength of all connective tissue. Such symptoms of premature aging as wrinkles and flabby skin can be brought about by weak collagen as a result of vitamin C deficiency.

Vitamin C is linked to the health and proper functioning of the adrenal glands. It assists in the oxygenation of cells. Vitamin C can help you fight infections, protect you against stress and fatigue, promote healing. It shortens post-operative convalescence. Heavy doses of vitamin C, 500 to 1,000 milligrams every two hours, can nip an approaching cold in the bud and prevent its development.

Dr. W. J. McCormick, the greatest authority on vitamin C in the world, has used large doses to treat patients with acute poisoning. Vitamin C can help to protect you from the harmful effect of poisons in your food and your environment. Vitamin C should be taken whenever medication is prescribed as it counteracts the adverse effects of most drugs.

A deficiency of vitamin C can age you prematurely and rob you of zest for living. It will cause cellular oxidation-reduction, fragility of blood vessels and capillaries and lowered resistance to all infections.

The best natural sources of vitamin C are fresh fruits and vegetables, such as oranges, grapefruit, strawberries, apples, broccoli, green peppers, turnip greens, etc. The best source of all is rose hips. Rose hips, which contain twenty to forty times more vitamin C than oranges, are the fruits of the rose. The best hip-bearing wild varieties of the rose are grown in Scandinavian countries, and imported Scandinavian rose hips are sold in every health food store in the United States.

Natural vitamin C has greater biological value than pure synthetic white tablets of ascorbic acid. Natural vitamin C is made from rose hips or other vegetable sources, which also contain other C-complex factors, such as rutin, citrin, and hesperidin. But in cases of acute infections and disease, when large doses of vitamin C are needed, a pure drug-store variety of vitamin C, ascorbic acid, may be used, preferably in combination with fresh orange, grapefruit or lemon juice. Vitamin C is completely harmless even when taken in huge amounts. Also keep in mind that vitamin C cannot be stored in the body for any appreciable length of time; the supplies in excess of immediate needs are excreted, so you must replace it daily.

The official recommended daily intake is set at 70 milligrams which is considered by many authorities as far too low. In view of the paramount role that the vitamin plays; and because of its general health-protective and disease-fighting property; and also because the vitamin C content of our foods is diminishing each year, we should all take extra vitamin C supplement each day. The vitamin C content in fruits and vegetables dwindles rapidly after harvesting. Most of us cannot obtain really fresh fruits and vegetables (although with modern transportation and merchandising methods they *look* fresh for months). Nationwide tests show that vitamin C is the most deficient element in the American diet. Many authorities today recommend doses of 200 and 300 milligrams a day of vitamin C as preventive measure, and 1,000 to 2,000 milligrams in acute infections or other conditions of ill health.

HOW TO FORTIFY YOUR DIET WITH VITAMIN C

1. Eat lots of fresh, raw fruit and vegetables every day.
2. Drink at least one glass of freshly made vegetable or fruit juice each day.
3. Use potent rose hip tablets and/or drink rose hip tea, as they do in Scandinavian countries. Rose hip tablets, powder or tea are sold in every health food store.
4. In times of stress, colds, infections and fatigue, take extra amounts of vitamin C in tablet form.

VITAMIN D

The best-known function of vitamin D is to assist in assimilation of calcium and phosphorus from the intestinal tract. These minerals are indispensible for all body functions, but particularly for bone building. Calcium deficiencies are common, particularly in older people, mainly because of malabsorption. Severe deficiency of vitamin D causes rickets in children, although the diet may have sufficient amounts of bone-building minerals.

Vitamin D also influences the parathyroid glands, which regulate the calcium level in the blood, and the thyroid which controls the metabolic rate of the cells. Other symptoms of vitamin D deficiency are nervousness, muscular fatigue, tooth decay, constipation and disposition to osteo-arthritis in older people.

Vitamin D is scarce in most foods. It is manufactured through the body's exposure to sunshine. Under the influence of the sun's rays, *ergosterol,* or vitamin D, is produced in the skin. Butter, milk, fish, eggs and mushrooms contain some vitamin D, but the amounts are small. The best natural dietary source of vitamin D is fish liver oil; cod liver oil and halibut oil are most commonly used. Halibut oil contains five to ten times more vitamin D than cod liver oil.

If you are exposed to the sunlight reasonably often, you probably have enough vitamin D. Those who are not exposed, especially during the winter months, should fortify their diets with a daily dose of fish liver oil. The minimum daily requirement is 400 to 800 units. Read the label and take a sufficient amount. Children should take fish liver oil routinely in the winter time.

Fish liver oils are high on the list of virility foods mainly because of their enormous amount of vitamin A, which is important for the health of testicular tissue and all mucous linings, including those of the sexual organs.

VITAMIN E

Vitamin E is known by the following pet names: "reproductive vitamin", "anti-sterility vitamin", "anti-abortion vitamin"; and in Sweden and Russia it is simply called "the sex vitamin." In the United States, long inhibited by pseudo-prudishness toward sex, we hear of vitamin E as a "heart vitamin." Vitamin E has indeed been successfully used in the treatment of serious heart diseases, due to its oxygenating and anti-blood-clotting ability.

Vitamin E oxygenates the tissues and markedly reduces the need for oxygen intake. It has an anti-blood-clotting quality, which helps to prevent death through thrombosis or blood clot. It dilates blood vessels and prevents excessive scar tissue production. These properties are extremely important in heart attacks when part of the heart tissue is destroyed. Vitamin E is the best aid a "heart case" can have.

In the context of this book, vitamin E is closely involved in many reproductive and sexual functions. A serious deficiency of vitamin E causes degeneration of the epithelial or germinal cells of the testicles. Vitamin E also protects sex hormones from destruction by oxidation. In the female, vitamin E has been prescribed in an attempt to prevent miscarriages and stillbirths. Dr. Evan Shute, of Shute Clinic in London, Ontario, a leading pioneer in clinical use of the vitamin, has used vitamin E extensively and successfully in the treatment of male sterility, miscarriages and menopausal symptoms. In one study he used vitamin E on 153 pregnancies in which there were 122 threatened abortions and 87 threatened miscarriages. 60 percent of the abortions and 86 percent of the miscarriages were prevented by vitamin E treatment. Dr. Shute says that vitamin E deficiency is very common in pregnant women.

A Hungarian doctor has found that vitamin E decreases pain in childbirth labor. Also, vitamin E relieves the symptoms of menopause such as hot flashes and dizziness. Doctors usually prescribe doses of 150 to 300 International Units a day in such cases.

The best natural sources of vitamin E are wheat germ

and wheat germ oil. Other good sources are corn oil, soy oil, cottonseed oil, sunflower oil. Green vegetables are also good sources, particularly cauliflower, spinach, brussels sprouts and kale. Milk and dairy products are reasonably good sources. Vitamin E may be obtained in capsule form from a drug store or health food store. Ask your doctor for the dosage proper for you.

HOW TO FORTIFY YOUR DIET WITH VITAMIN E

1. Take one or two teaspoons of wheat germ oil each day (or take wheat germ oil capsules).

2. Use two or three tablespoons of fresh, raw wheat germ each day. It can be sprinkled over cereals or mixed with juices or milk. A word of caution—old, rancid wheat germ is not only useless, it is also definitely harmful. In European health food stores wheat germ is dated to indicate the time of production and packaging. Although I have given frequent recommendations for health food products in this book, I must say that I have yet to find fresh edible raw wheat germ in an American health food store. Never buy raw wheat germ without first tasting it. If it leaves a bitter taste in your mouth after chewing, don't buy it. It will do you more harm than good.

Before we leave vitamin E, let me tell of a striking case of vitamin E therapy that I have witnessed. A good friend of mine in Canada, Mrs. K., had seven early miscarriages during eight years of childless marriage. For several years I admonished her to try wheat germ oil and vitamin E, but her obstetrician did not think the advice worth considering. Mrs. K. decided to try it when another friend of hers, a veterinarian, told her that my prescription was identical with one he had been using successfully on cows and horses to prevent miscarriages. Within three months she became pregnant and, after a full nine-month pregnancy, delivered a perfectly healthy boy. By the way, her husband took raw wheat germ and wheat germ oil, too.

VITAMIN F

Vitamin F is more commonly known as *essential fatty acids*. Vitamin F is extremely important in many vital body functions. Here are some examples:

- It is necessary for normal glandular activity, especially of the adrenal glands.
- It is essential for the prevention of cholestrol deposits in the arteries.
- It protects you against the harmful effects of x-rays.
- It promotes availability of calcium to the cells.
- It is important for healthy skin and for prevention of such disorders as eczema, allergies, asthma, colds and sinus infections.

Professor P. A. Owren, of Oslo University in Norway, has found that *linolenic acid,* one of the essential fatty acids found in vegetable oils, can prevent heart attacks caused by blood clot. Linseed oil and soybean oil are the richest sources of linolenic acid.

Vitamin F has been also used in treatment of prostate disorders and menstrual disturbance.

The richest natural sources of vitamin F are cold-pressed, unrefined vegetable oils: wheat germ oil, linseed oil, sunflower oil, safflower oil and soybean oil. Use these oils generously in salads and for general cooking purposes. Do not use hardened, or hydrogenated fats such as margarine and solid shortenings. In the process of hydrogenation the essential fatty acids have been destroyed.

VITAMIN K

Vitamin K maintains the blood level of *prothrombin,* one of the factors essential for blood coagulation. Massive doses of vitamins K and C have been helpful in the treatment of stubborn nosebleeds. A deficiency of vitamin K may cause hemorrhages in any part of the body.

The best sources of vitamin K are green leafy vegetables. One of the richest is kelp, or seaweed. Much research has been done on seaweed in Japan. A Japanese doctor, Shichiro Goto, M.D., says that seaweed contains large amounts of vitamin K, and that vitamin K is essential for liver activity, adrenal function, heart and kidney function. He claims that vitamin K is an important vitality and longevity factor. Don't forget that bird nest soup, famous for its virility-increasing property, is made largely of seaweed.

VITAMIN P

Vitamin P is better known in the United States as *bioflavonoids.* There is much controversy in regard to vitamin P. The FDA claims it is an ineffective and worthless substance. However, much European research, particularly in Russia, has demonstrated otherwise. Vitamin P is reported to have been successfully used in the treatment of hemorrhoids, respiratory infections, high blood pressure, varicose veins, habitual abortions, rheumatic fever, anemia and damage caused by x-rays.

The main property of vitamin P is its ability to increase the strength of the capillaries and regulate their permeability (P stands for permeability). Vitamin P also assists vitamin C in keeping the collagen in a healthy condition. Vitamins P and C are *synergists*—

i.e. the combined effect of both substances administered together is greater than the sum of the individual effects. It may be that some of the research done in the United States, which was unfavorable to the effectiveness of vitamin P, was incomplete and misleading because the synergistic effect of vitamins C and P was not taken into consideration.

The best sources of vitamin P, or bioflavonoids, are fresh raw fruits and vegetables. Citrus fruits, green peppers, apricots, grapes, apples, strawberries and black currants are especially rich in vitamin P. Rose hips are the richest natural source of vitamin C and also an excellent source of vitamin P. Try to have ample fresh fruits and rose hips in your diet.

MINERALS

Minerals are as important as vitamins. Sufficient amounts of minerals are needed to assure sound bones and muscles, steady nerves and a keen mind. Minerals are also needed for the healthy function of your endocrine and sex glands.

CALCIUM is essential for all the vital functions of your body. Without enough calcium your bones become brittle, your nerves jittery, your muscles flabby. Nervousness, mental depression and insomnia are other symptoms of calcium deficiency. Calcium is needed for the proper clotting of blood to prevent muscular cramps and to speed the healing process.

The best sources of calcium are milk and cheese, and most raw vegetables, such as endive, lettuce, cauliflower, cabbage, dandelion greens, kale, watercress, Brussels sprouts, broccoli and tomatoes. Other excellent sources are sesame seeds, oats, navy beans, almonds, walnuts, millet, brown rice, wheat germ and sunflower seeds. Sesame seeds are extremely rich in calcium. They contain almost twice as much calcium as phosphorus; other grains are deficient in calcium and high in phosphorus.

PHOSPHORUS is a mineral colleague of calcium. They work together and must be in proper balance to be effective. Phosphorus is needed for healthy nerves and for mental work. It is also a factor in carbohydrate metabolism and in the acid-alkaline balance of the blood and tissues.

A phosphorus deficiency may result in retarded growth, reduced sexual powers, general weakness, poor bone development and deficient nerve and brain function. The old belief that "fish is good for the brain" may have some scientific justification. Fish is rich in phosphorus that is essential for brain cells.

The best food sources of phosphorus are dairy products, egg yolks, fish, whole grains, nuts, seeds and beans, oranges, grapefruit, apples, asparagus, celery, lettuce, cauliflower, olives, corn, watercress, artichokes, broccoli, cabbage, carrots and avocados.

IRON is needed to supply all the cells of your body with oxygen. An iron deficiency will cause anemia. Needless to say, an anemic person is a poor lover. Iron is essential for the production of *hemoglobin,* which carries the oxygen from your lungs to every cell of your body. The importance of good oxygenation cannot be overemphasized. Plenty of iron is needed in your blood to make you energetic and virile—in work and play. Iron deficiency can cause a lowered resistance to disease, general rundown feeling, shortness of breath in exercise, headaches, poor complexion and low interest in sex.

Iron deficiencies are common in women of reproductive age who have an abundant menstrual flow. Recent studies showed that in *two-thirds* of women of child-bearing age and in the *majority* of pregnant women, the body stores of iron were low or absent. This study prompted the recent action by the Food and Nutrition Board to increase the recommended dietary allowance for iron from 15 to 18 milligrams per day for women from ten to fifty-five. Iron deficiencies in American children are only too common. A recent survey, conducted by the U.S. Public Health Service, revealed a shocking picture—one-third of all children under six are anemic!

The best dietary sources of iron are turnip greens, wheat germ, brewer's yeast, liver, dark molasses, beet tops, spinach, dates, apricots, peaches, prunes, raisins, beans, peas and nuts. Brewer's yeast is rich in iron, in addition to its storehouse of B-complex vitamins and proteins.

A sufficient amount of gastric enzymes, especially of hydrocholoric acid, is needed for proper digestion and assimilation of iron. Older people are often anemic in spite of plentiful iron in their diet, because they lack sufficient hydrochloric acid in their stomachs. For these reasons, the iron-containing fruits are the most reliable sources of dietary iron. Apricots are particularly rich in iron. Fruits, when eaten raw, contain their own enzymes and acids which help the body to release the iron and utilize it. The best protection against iron deficiency is to avoid all refined foods and eat lots of raw fruits and vegetables.

COPPER is similar to iron in its action. Iron cannot be absorbed without copper. Copper is involved in hemoglobin production, protein metabolism, in healing processes, and perhaps in keeping the natural color of the hair.

Foods rich in copper are generally those rich in iron. Especially good sources are almonds, beans, peas, whole wheat products, prunes and pomegranate.

IODINE is an extremely important trace element. *Thyroxin,* the thyroid hormone which regulates much of your physical and mental activity is made almost totally of iodine and amino acids.

Iodine deficiency in a diet may cause goiter and enlargement of the thyroid gland, or exophthalmic goiter, also called toxic goiter. It may also cause nervous disturbances, hair loss and fading, susceptibility to infections, overweight, sterility, lowered mental activity and generally lowered stamina.

Iodine-deficient soil is the main reason for dietary iodine deficiency. The soils in the Great Lakes region and the North Central States are deficient in iodine, which results in iodine-deficient foods. Iodinized salt is a good protection against iodine deficiencies, but eating too much salt is not advisable; therefore the best iodine supplement is kelp, or seaweed tablets. One or two kelp tablets a day will supply you with a daily requirement of iodine.

The other dietary sources of iodine are: pineapples, pears, artichokes, citrus fruits, watercress, and, of course, seafood. Sea water is a good source of iodine. Use sea salt instead of ordinary salt. If you live close to the sea, why not take a tablespoon or two of sea water each day? Provided, of course, that the local water is not polluted. Sea water is a fabulous source of all the beneficial minerals and trace elements, including iodine.

POTASSIUM is important for normal heartbeat. It also promotes the secretion of hormones and helps the kidneys in their detoxicative work. It is considered of special importance for the prevention of female disorders because of its stimulating influence on the endocrine hormone production. Dr. P. E. Formica of New Jersey, has treated what he calls "the housewife syndrome" defined as chronic fatigue, insomnia and lethargy in relation to housework and lovemaking, with a prescription drug which contains potassium, magnesium and aspartic acid. Eighty-seven percent of the housewives responded favorably.[4]

---

[4] Taub, Harold J., The Eight Foods that Spark Sexual Desire, *Pageant*, April, 1966

Potassium helps to excrete excessive amounts of salt from the tissues and is essential for healthy muscle tone. A deficiency of potassium can cause muscle weakness in every part of the body, extreme fatigue and constipation. It has been demonstrated in animal tests that potassium deficiency can be one of the causes of high blood pressure.

The best sources of potassium are potatoes (potato peelings contain most of the potassium—so don't throw them away!), most green leafy vegetables, whole grain breads and cereals, nuts, most fruits, milk and cheese.

SODIUM is, of course, salt. It is needed in the body for many vital functions. But most people eat more salt than is good for them. You actually need only 0.2 to 0.6 grams of salt a day. This amount can be easily obtained from any diet of natural foods, without the addition of extra salt. Over five grams of salt a day is considered harmful. Many people eat as much as ten to fifteen grams a day. It has been demonstrated that too much salt can cause high blood pressure, loss of hair, and possibly rheumatic conditions. The assumption that we "lose" salt in perspiration is erroneous and without scientific support. The body uses sweating as a welcome chance to throw out unwanted deposits of salt from the tissues. An excessive consumption of salt leads to water retention in the tissues and is a contributing cause of premature aging.

If you like salt, use sea salt moderately. Sea salt contains most other valuable minerals as well as sodium. Sea salt is sold in health food stores.

CHLORINE helps the liver in its detoxicating activity; and is essential for the production of hydrochloric acid which is needed in the stomach, for the proper digestion of proteins and for mineral assimilation.

The best sources of chlorine are: seaweed (kelp), watercress, avocado, chard, tomatoes, cabbage, endive, cucumbers, asparagus, pineapple, cherries, oats, wheat germ, milk and salt-water fish.

MAGNESIUM is a "new" mineral in the sense that its extraordinary importance in human nutrition has been newly reemphasized. Magnesium activates certain enzymes and helps in utilization of calcium and other minerals. It is needed for healthy muscle tone and may be capable of preventing premature wrinkles.

The best sources of magnesium: figs, lemons, apples, peaches, grapefruit, raspberries, endive, lettuce, cauliflower, celery, almonds, whole grains, sunflower seeds, brown rice and sesame seeds.

SULPHUR, the "beauty mineral," is essential for healthy hair, skin and nails.

The best sources are: radishes, turnips, onions, celery, string beans, horseradish, watercress and kale.

MANGANESE is a trace element needed in minute quantity. That quantity nevertheless is extremely important to the proper coordinative action between the brain and the nerves and muscles in every part of the body. Manganese is also involved in normal reproduction and the propert function of mammary glands.

The best food sources are: oranges and grapefruit, apricots, green leafy vegetables, the outer coatings of nuts and grains, kelp, raw egg yolk and salt-water fish.

SILICON is especially beneficial in healing processes, healthy growth of teeth, hair and nails. The best sources: steel-cut oats, apples, strawberries, grapes, beets, onions, parsnips and other vegetables.

FLUORINE is needed for bone-building. It also acts as an internal antiseptic; it protects against infections. *Organic flourine* is found in steel-cut oats, sunflower seeds, milk and cheese, garlic, green vegetables and sea water.

ZINC is of specific importance in the context of this book. It is essential for healthy sex organs and for the normal function of the prostate gland. There is high concentration of zinc in sperm, seminal fluid and in the prostate itself, more than in any other part of the body. Deficiency in zinc according to some authorities is a probable cause of enlargement of the prostate and other unhealthy changes in this important sex gland. This is specifically important to men past middle age, when prostate troubles usually start. Zinc deficiency is also associated with retarded development of sexual organs, or hypogonadism.

The best natural sources of zinc are: wheat bran and wheat germ, brewer's yeast, milk, eggs, onions, oysters, pumpkin seeds and sunflower seeds. Pumpkin seeds and sunflower seeds are especially rich sources of zinc.

Other important trace elements are *COBALT, BROMINE, NICKEL, LITHIUM, BORON.*

HOW TO GET A MAXIMUM OF VITAMINS, MINERALS AND TRACE ELEMENTS IN YOUR DIET

It is important to realize that vitamins, minerals, enzymes, trace elements, amino acids, fatty acids and other nutritive substances all work together as a team, helping one another in various processes in your body. When this totality is disturbed, when some nutrients are oversupplied and others undersupplied, the life rhythm is upset and health disturbances of various kinds will set in. When you eat *natural, whole, unrefined,* and *unprocessed* foods, you can rest assured that you will receive *all* their vital nutrients in the proper balance. When you eat refined, cooked, processed foods, the vitamin and mineral balance is disturbed and you will invariably obtain too little of some substances, comparatively too much of others and perhaps none of another group. Here are a few examples:

- In refining and processing of wheat, most minerals are removed.
- Cooking vegetables in water likewise leaches minerals out.
- Cooking removes or destroys much of vitamins C and B.

- Food processing removes most of vitamin E from grains where it is normally abundant.

Therefore, the best way to assure that you are getting all the vitamins, minerals, enzymes and trace elements in your diet is to eat *natural foods*. Eat most of your food raw. Fresh raw vegetables and fruits, whole grains, seeds and nuts, milk, cheese, eggs and vegetable oils are full of all the vitamins, minerals, proteins, fatty acids, enzymes and trace elements you need for optimum health and sexual virility.

Final note: overeating and obesity are destroyers of virility. Obesity is largely caused by devitalized, nutritionless foods. Although you eat a lot you still feel hungry because the devitalized foods are lacking the nutrients you so desperately need. So you eat more and grow fatter and fatter. In other words, you are *overfed but undernourished*. When you start to eat natural foods, which are filled with all the nutrients nature put in them, you will be satisfied with less food. You can even be *underfed and well-nourished* at the same time on nutrition-packed natural, whole, unrefined foods. And your vitality, longevity—and virility—will increase with every inch of unnecessary fat that you shed from your waist!

VITAL POINTS IN CHAPTER 10

1. Vitamins, minerals, and trace elements are absolutely essential for your health and optimum vitality.
2. Directly and indirectly, vitamins and minerals are vitally involved in your sexual health and reproductive capacity.
3. Description of most common vitamins and minerals and trace elements, and how and where to obtain them.
4. How to fortify your diet with special food supplements to assure a plentiful supply of all the important vitamins and minerals.

CHAPTER 11

TEN SPECIAL FOODS TO MAINTAIN AND ENHANCE YOUR SEXUAL VIGOR

FROM THE PRECEDING chapters you have learned that the basis for a healthy and happy sex life lies in optimal nutrition. Nutrition is *not* the whole answer, of course, and in itself cannot guarantee sexual contentment, because so many other factors may be involved. But the fact remains that your sexual health and physical capacity for love are closely tied to the state of your health generally and your endocrine and sex glands in particular; and that the quality of your health and the efficiency of your glandular functions depend largely on adequate and proper nutrition. *Nutrition is the most important single factor affecting not only your physical health, but also your mental health.*

Optimal nutrition will have a favorable stabilizing effect on your mental and psychological responses and your total emotional equilibrium, thus helping to eliminate some of the non-organic psychic factors connected with sexual disorders and impotence. Any way you look at it, nutrition plays a vital part in your sexual health. A. C. Kinsey, Havelock Ellis, Th.H. Van de Velde, William J. Robinson and other giants of modern science who have delved into the study, have all noted that nutrition plays a not inconsiderable part in frequency and nature of human sexual activity.

Dr. George Belham said, "The essence of potency is healthy sensible eating, reinforced by particular factors that have a reasonable basis for their claim to enhance virility and help overcome impotence."[1]

"SPECIAL" FOODS FOR SEXUAL VIGOR

In addition to foods which possess general health-promoting qualities, special food substances are discussed in this chapter which have a particular effect on maintaining and enhancing your sexual vigor. These foods *are not aphrodisiacs. They are all completely natural and harmless foods.* They will not overstimulate your sexual glands and endanger your health, but will help your glands to reach a *peak of healthy activity.*

Seven of the ten special foods have been used for thousands of years for the purpose of enhancing amatory prowess. These are: honey, milk, eggs, sesame seeds, raw nuts and seeds, kelp (bird nest soup) and fish liver oil. They are named and recommended in many ancient writings and recipes. They have been handed down from generation to generation. Their reputations are time-tested.

The remaining three—wheat germ, wheat germ oil, and lecithin—are more recent foods, which were unknown to the ancients. Although vegetable oils have been pressed from seeds for several thousand years, the ancients lacked the capacity to extract oil from wheat. Wheat has been, of course, used as a food (even as an aphrodisiac food) for thousands of years, but the separation of the germ and

---

[1] Belham, George, THE VIRILITY DIET, Dell Publishing Co., Inc., New York, 1968. Copyright (c) 1965 by George Belham

the extraction of oil from it are relatively recent inventions. Lecithin is also a very recent food. First discovered in eggs at the end of the last century, lecithin, as a mass-production food, has been available only for a few decades. It is made from soybeans and is available at all health food stores.

1. WHEAT GERM

Wheat has always been one of the staple foods. In many cultures, wheat has been a symbol of health and fertility. Ancient writings often named bread as an aphrodisiac food. In some nations—Russia, Bulgaria, Finland, to name a few—bread constitutes a major part of the daily diet.

Wheat is one of the most nutritious substances known to man. Packed with vitamins, minerals, fatty acids and proteins, it is a powerful source of energy and health.

Man seems to go out of his way, using ingenuity and inventiveness, to destroy and spoil his food before he eats it. It would be difficult to find a food which has been subjected to more spoilation than wheat. A century or so ago, man decided that his bread should be white instead of brown. He developed a milling process which could make beautifully white flour, resulting in snow-white bread. Why anyone should find white bread more beautiful than brown is hard to guess. The only rational explanation I know goes something like this:

> Man is a dumb and thoughtless fool:
> When it's hot he wants it cool;
> When it's cool, he wants it hot—
> *Always wanting what is not!*

With the same ostensible logic man changes the color of cheese from white to orange-yellow, or colors brown pecans red.

Once man had started his destructive campaign against his staple food, wheat, he didn't stop halfway. He did his job so thoroughly that he transformed a powerful health food, which was called the staff of life, into a worthless, nutritionless, tasteless, spongy white mass which goes on the supermarket shelf today under the name of bread. It is now stripped of virtually all the nutritive factors which made wheat such a treasured food for thousands of years. In the milling, refining and baking processes virtually all B-vitamins, unsaturated fatty acids and the all-important E vitamin—twenty-five known food factors—have been removed, together with most proteins and minerals. What remains is pure starch into which three synthetic B-vitamins and inorganic iron have been added.

The part of wheat which fared worst in this destructive process was *wheat germ.* It was totally removed for two reasons. It made flour darker; and flour spoiled faster because of the oil content of the wheat germ, which easily turned rancid in storage. So wheat germ was taken away from man's diet and sold for cattle feed.

As man changed from dark bread to white, his health started to deteriorate rapidly. Only much later, when vitamins B and E were discovered, was it apparent that by discarding the most nutritive part of the wheat, the germ, man deprived himself of the most potent source of these two vitamins in his diet. Serious deficiencies of these vitamins have been found to cause male and female sterility, among many other health disorders.

What is wheat germ? Germ is the part of a grain which is responsible for germinating or sprouting, and thus making a new plant. Germ carries the spark of new life, the reproductive capacity and life-generatiing power. It also contains all the nutritive substances, such as vitamins, proteins and minerals, necessary to nourish a new plant until it is able to feed itself from soil, water and air. Practically all of these vital nutrients are contained in germ and bran, which are the outer layers of the grain—and they are all removed in the refining process. White flour is made from endosperm, the white-colored center section of the wheat kernel, which is mostly starch.

But here is the tragicomical side of the situation. Truly, "one man's loss is another man's gain." Some smart people realized what a nutritional treasure wheat germ was and started to share its nutritional blessings with pigs, cattle and horses. Needless to say, farmers were overjoyed to have a cheap source of such powerful nutrition for their stock. They soon discovered that wheat germ made their animals healthier and stronger, that it increased both the conception rate of females and the reproductive power of males.

So wheat germ became the miracle health food of a few health-conscious people. It is now sold in health food stores and millions of people, including athletes and sportsmen enjoy its health-building and revitalizing power.

Why all this enthusiasm about wheat germ? And why should it be a part of high-virility diet?

Here are a few figures.

- A half cup of wheat germ contains 24 grams of protein—more than in a quarter pound of steak, and as much as in four eggs.
- Wheat germ is an excellent source of B-vitamins and vitamin E—both important for the health of the reproductive system.
- Wheat germ is one of the richest sources of iron.
- Wheat germ is a storehouse of minerals, especially phosphorus, manganese, magnesium, potassium, and copper.

As you can see, wheat germ *is* a wonder food! Take it as it is with milk and honey, sprinkle it on cereals and salads, or mix it with vegetable and fruit juices. It can be used in baking and cooking, or mixed in sauces.

Warning: raw wheat germ is perishable. Because of its rich vegetable oil content it turns rancid easily. This destroys the valuable vitamin E and makes it taste bitter.

Fresh, raw wheat germ should taste sweet. Insist on tasting before buying. If you can't get fresh wheat germ, buy toasted vacuum-packed wheat germ. Although toasting destroys some of the vitamins, it is still better than eating rancid wheat germ which is definitely harmful.

2. WHEAT GERM OIL

Wheat germ oil is the richest natural source of miracle vitamin E. Herbert Bailey, a noted medical writer, the author of the excellent book VITAMIN E: YOUR KEY TO A HEALTHY HEART, (Arc Books, 1967) calls vitamin E "the miracle of modern medicine," "one of the greatest medical discoveries of the century". There is hardly any condition of ill health that vitamin E will not affect favorably.

Vitamin E was discovered in 1922 in wheat germ oil. Since that time over seven hundred medical researches in seventeen countries have demonstrated the vitamin's extraordinary prophylactic and therapeutic value. In the context of this work we are limited by space to review only what is related to the health of the reproductive and sexual system, where vitamin E offers truly monumental benefits and hopes.

Here are a few things that vitamin E can do:

- Stimulate the production of sperm in the male.
- Prevent miscarriages and premature births.
- Provide effective aid to both male and female fertility.
- Prevent sterility in both sexes.
- Serve in the treatment of menopausal flashes and other menopausal disorders.
- Increase general vitality and muscular stamina by improving cardiac efficiency and by increasing tissue oxygenation.

The above-named properties of vitamin E are established by research. Here are a few dramatic examples.

Dr. R. Bayer, of West Germany, treated one hundred childless couples with vitamin E. More than half the couples had been able to conceive, but miscarriage had terminated all the pregnancies. After vitamin E treatments, the couples had seventy-nine pregnancies and only two women lost their babies. In a second group, in which repeated miscarriages were common, Dr. Bayer gave 100 milligrams of vitamin E to the men daily for one month before conception, and 200 milligrams daily for three months prior to conception to the wives. All the women conceived and forty-one pregnancies resulted in forty-one births of healthy offspring. Vitamin E proved to be not only a preventive against miscarriages but also an aid to fertility and to improvement of the sperm quality in the male.

Two American doctors, James B. Patterson and Wynne M. Silbernagel, reported that wheat germ oil, given to expectant mothers daily, reduced the number of premature babies by half.

Wheat germ oil has been long used by farmers to increase the reproductive power of livestock. Wheat germ oil reduces the risk of miscarriage, increases the conception rate and raises the reproductive power of male animals. As one Livestock Association manager said, "I suggest the use of wheat germ oil for slow-serving bulls; almost always the bull becomes normal within a month."

Vitamin E can markedly increase the sperm count in men and raise the volume of seminal fluid, as reported by Dr. E. Lindner. In a laboratory experiment with animals, sexual activity was induced and stimulated in both males and females by administration of wheat germ oil.[2]

A widespread deficiency of vitamin E has been noted

---

[2] *Endocrinology*, September, 1951

in the United States and other western countries. The Department of Agriculture reported in 1965 that some people have a "dangerously low blood level of vitamin E." One of the main reasons for this is, of course, that vitamin E has been largely removed from foods by processing. Wheat is one of the best sources of vitamin E, but wheat germ, containing vitamin E, has been refined out of our bread. You would have to eat ten loaves of white bread daily for minimum requirement of this vitamin.

How much vitamin E do you need to protect yourself from disorders in the reproductive system and assure a high level of sexual vigor and health? Dr. Evan Shute, the world's foremost authority on vitamin E, maintains that the bare minimum should be 100 International Units a day. He recommends twice that much for a margin of safety.

You will be in no danger of overdosage if you obtain your vitamin E from wheat germ oil. Another point—some researchers are not sure what substances in wheat germ oil have such a miraculous effect on the health of the reproductive system. In some experiments, a synthetic vitamin E was not able to duplicate the results obtained by wheat germ oil. The doctors feel that wheat germ oil may contain other active factors as yet undiscovered. You can benefit from these mystery factors when you take wheat germ oil instead of a synthetic vitamin E capsule. You can buy wheat germ oil in capsules or liquid form from health food stores.

Wheat germ oil is the richest natural source of vitamin E—as high as 420 I.U. per 100 grams. Other food sources of vitamin E are: rice germ oil, sunflower seed oil, safflower oil, peanut oil, cottonseed oil, wheat germ, raw walnuts, filberts, almonds, cabbage, parsley, turnip greens and sweet potatoes.

Severe vitamin E deficiency can cause degeneration and atrophy of the testes, diminished sex hormone production and sterility. If wheat germ oil can prevent and correct these conditions, why not make it a part of your daily virility diet?

3. SESAME SEEDS

Sesame, cultivated by man for thousands of years, is often named in ancient writings as a powerful virility food. Sesame is used widely in Africa, and the Middle and Far East. In India and China sesame is a staple food. Armenian Turks use it in a liquid form called *Matahini,* which is a respected rejuvenator of mental and physical capacities and endurance. In Israel, Turkey and Arabian countries, *Halvah,* a candy made of sesame and honey, is very popular. The women of ancient Babylonia used Halvah to enhance their sex appeal and to restore their men's virility. Halvah is sold in health food stores in the United States and also in New York's old-country type markets.

Sesame may have been brought to this country from Africa and sesame cakes are still used in parts of the South. In South America, sesame seed oil is called "the Queen of the Oils," because of its extraordinary cosmetic properties. Health food stores also sell a butterlike spread made from sesame seeds, called *Tahini.*

Sesame seeds are richer in calcium than milk, cheese or nuts. Their protein content is 19 to 28 per cent—higher than that of meat; sesame seed protein is high in quality. Sesame is an especially good source of the important amino acid *methionine,* which is otherwise scarce in proteins of vegetable source. The seeds are rich in unsaturated fatty acids—55 per cent of the seed is oil. The content is high in B-vitamins, niacin, inositol and choline, and vitamin E.

Sesame is also an excellent source of lecithin, an organic phosphorized fat which is a chief constituent of brain and nerve tissue, and an essential component of semen. The concentration of lecithin in the master gland pituitary and in the pineal is higher than in any other part of the body. Lecithin is an effective aid in keeping your blood vessels functional, free from cholesterol deposits. (See section on lecithin in this chapter.)

The value of sesame seeds, particularly in the form of halvah, as aphrodisiac food, was supported by a French doctor's research a few years ago. Sesame seeds have abundant magnesium and potassium, and honey is rich in aspartic acid, one of the amino acids. Some doctors have used a very similar prescription formula—the potassium and magnesium salts of aspartic acid—to treat women with "the housewife syndrome" or chronic fatigue, insomnia and lethargy in lovemaking. Eighty-seven per cent responded with a startling change in condition.

Here is how you can use sesame in your kitchen. Buy some sesame seeds from your health food store. Sprinkle them on cereals, use them in baking. Sesame seeds are used on top of some rolls and French bread sold in the United States. Or grind them in your seed grinder (obtainable from department stores for about ten dollars) and mix with honey to make halvah—see recipe below. The Romans had an old custom of giving soldiers an emergency ration—cakes made of sesame seeds and honey. Experience had convinced them that man could walk farther and survive longer on this ration than on any other food of equal weight. You can also buy Tahini and use it as you would peanut butter, or mix it with water in a blender for sesame milk. Sesame seed oil is wonderful on salads.

Here is the recipe for homemade halvah:

HALVAH

1 cup sesame seeds
2 tsp. coagulated, natural honey.

Grind sesame seeds in an electric seed grinder. Pour sesame meal in a large cup and knead honey into it with a large spoon until honey is well mixed and halvah acquires the consistency of hard dough. Serve it as it is, or make small balls and roll them in whole sesame seeds, shredded coconut, sunflower seeds or wheat germ—and enjoy one of the finest and best tasting health and virility foods in the world!

4. HONEY

As you have seen from the review of the ancient aphrodisiacs in Chapter 7, honey has always been regarded as a potent aphrodisiac. Why does honey have this reputation?

Since time immemorial man has regarded honey as ambrosia—a food of the gods. The Bible mentions and praises honey countless times. Neolithic cave paintings illustrated honeycombs collected for food about fifteen thousand years ago. Three-thousand-year old honey has been found in Egyptian pyramids—still edible and with its characteristic aroma preserved. The great physicians of old, Pythagoras, Hippocrates and others, recommended honey as a revitalizing and rejuvenating food.

Recently, Russian scientists have made a study of the eating habits of their centenarians. They found that *all* persons over one hundred were using honey as a principle food in their diet. Many were beekeepers. Russian scientists report that pollen is probably the active substance in honey responsible for its rejuvenating property. Pollen is the male germ cells which are collected from flowers by bees and deposited in honey. Natural, unstrained and unrefined honey contains large amounts of pollen, but the refined, clarified supermarket-type of honey is largely free from it.

Pollen seems to be the most complete food in nature. It

contains twenty per cent complete proteins, all the water soluble vitamins, especially B and C, and plenty of minerals, enzymes and trace elements. Pollen also contains a *gonadotropic hormone,* a plant hormone which is similar to the pituitary hormone *gonadotropin,* which stimulates the sex glands. Pollen has been used by researchers for the treatment of gastric disorders, asthma, hay fever and prostate troubles. A Swedish authority, Professor Ask-Upmark, cured acute prostate inflammations with pollen preparations.

Honey has been used both as food and medicine throughout the ages. In addition to its definite age-retarding property, honey is known to be effective in the following conditions:

- It increases calcium retention in the system.
- It increases hemoglobin count and can prevent or cure nutritional anemia. It is rich in iron and copper.
- It is beneficial in the treatment of liver and kidney disorders, diseases of the respiratory and digestive tract, colds, poor circulation and bad complexion.
- It strengthens heart action and is especially beneficial for old people.
- It is an excellent bacteria-destroying agent: it speeds the healing processes of ulcers and sores.

Honey indeed fulfills more than any other food, Hippocrates' requirement for an ideal food: "Our food must be our medicine—our medicine must be our food."

Honey as a food is vastly superior to white sugar. Whereas sugar is completely devoid of nutritional value, with the exception of chemically pure carbohydrates, natural honey is an extremely nutritious food. Its sugars are in a predigested form and are quickly absorbed by the bloodstream. Easily obtainable sugar is vital for many important body functions, including the manufacture of male seminal fluid, of which sugar is an important element. Lack of sufficient glycogen in the system will slow down or reduce the production of semen and thus dampen amorous desires. Honey is an excellent source of sugars which are easily and very quickly converted into glycogen.

Some doctors believe that the active factor in honey is aspartic acid. The salts of aspartic acid have been used to treat chronic fatigue, insomnia and lethargy in relation to housework and lovemaking. Sesame seeds and honey are the ingredients in halvah, an ancient food used to enhance sex appeal.

Important note: Use only raw, natural, unstrained, and unpasteurized honey. Heating destroys both vitamins and enzymes. Refining, filtering and "clarifying" of honey removes minerals and amino acids, including aspartic acid, and—what is even worse—removes all the pollen. Always choose the darker varieties of honey, which contain more minerals and vitamins.

Honey is a nature's miracle food which will keep you feeling younger longer. Science has not been able to pinpoint the exact factors in honey responsible for its supposed rejuvenating and revitalizing properties—3.73 per cent of honey is still so-called "undetermined matter" which does not yield to analysis. The real rejuvenating power of honey may be in that elusive 3.73 percent.

5. RAW NUTS AND SEEDS

Nuts, seeds and grains are the most potent of all foods. They contain the secret of life itself, the germ. This spark of life is of extreme importance for man's life, his health and his virility.

> "And God said, Behold, I have given you every herb bearing seed, which is upon the face of the

earth, and every tree, in which is the fruit of a tree yielding seed; to you it shall be for meat."

Genesis, 1:29

The nutritional power of seeds is fantastic. Here is just a glimpse:

- Seeds, grains, and nuts are gold mines of minerals.
- They contain most of the vitamins, especially vitamins B, E, and F.
- They are excellent sources of proteins. Although most grain proteins are not "complete," they are valuable nevertheless, particularly in combination with vegetables, milk, or eggs.

Phosphorus has been reputed throughout the ages both as a brain mineral and a virility mineral. The popularity of fish as a brain food is based on its high content of phosphorus. Although no definite research has substantiated these claims, we do know that phosphorus is an extremely important factor in the efficient functioning of both brain and nerves; and that phosphorus is involved in sugar metabolism, which is vitally linked with the sex drive. Seeds, grains, and nuts are the best food sources of phosphorus.

In a high-virility diet raw nuts, seeds and grain foods are particularly important for two reasons:

1. *B-vitamin and minerals.* Proper sugar metabolism is imperative for optimal sexual power. Your body cannot use the various forms of sugar and carbohydrates you supply with food. It must convert them into a useable form of sugar called *glycogen*, which can be stored in the body and used as needed.

Glycogen is vitally involved, for instance, in production of seminal fluid. To change food carbohydrates into glycogen, your body sets up a complex chemical process, in which various enzymes, vitamins and minerals are involved. Ample amounts of B-complex vitamins, especially thiamine, are needed to digest and transform the carbohydrates. Magnesium, potassium, and phosphorus are also indispensible in the process. If any of these substances are missing, as they are in refined carbohydrates, the process of sugar conversion will be disturbed. The deficiency may show up in reduced production of semen. (This may explain the folklore belief in the aphrodisiac value of snails. Snails are the only known food that contains pure glycogen.)

Seeds, nuts and whole grains are abundant sources of B-complex vitamins and minerals, necessary for the efficient quick conversion of sugars into glycogen.

2. *Zinc*. There are more than five million infertile husbands in the United States, and an even higher number of partially fertile males. Also, prostate troubles have been steadily on the increase. Until recently, medical science could not give a satisfactory explanation for these problems. Now, however, several studies indicate that deficiency of the trace mineral, *zinc*, may be associated both with the prostate disorders and with dwindling fertility.

Medical researchers have found that in Iran and Egypt, where many people have zinc deficient diets, many boys suffer from retarded development of the gonads. When the diet is supplemented with zinc, they quickly mature sexually. A very high concentration of zinc has been found in the sperm, seminal fluid and the prostate itself: in fact there is more zinc in the prostate gland than in any other part of the body. A deficiency of zinc can cause enlargement and other unhealthy changes in this vital sex gland. Two recent laboratory investigations showed that the main difference between healthy and diseased prostate glands is the amount of zinc in the tissue. Scientists are convinced that deficiency of zinc is closely related to prostate deterioration.

Is it possible to have a deficiency of zinc on a normal "well-balanced" diet? Yes, if you eat average American meals. Zinc is virtually non-existant in refined, processed foods. The best sources of zinc are whole grains and seeds. When bran and germ are removed from grains, zinc is taken out, too. In addition, the minerals in your food can come only from the soil; but the soils of thirty-two out of fifty states are deficient in zinc. So your food is deficient in zinc to start with.

Foods rich in zinc are whole grains, wheat bran, wheat germ, brewer's yeast, oysters, herring, eggs and onions. Sunflower seeds and pumpkin seeds are excellent sources of zinc.

A German doctor discovered that in certain countries where pumpkin seeds are eaten regularly and in great quantities, there is virtually no incidence of prostate trouble. Dr. Bela Pater, of Klausenburg, believes that in addition to zinc and other excellent nutritive qualities, pumpkin seeds contain a "plant hormone" which affects man's hormone production, in part by substitution and in part by proliferation.

The International Society for Research on Nutrition and Vital Substances recommends the cereal products, prepared from whole grains and seeds, as the basis of a macrobiotic diet. Macrobiotics, of course, is *the art of living longer while enjoying better health.*

In addition to such widely distributed grain and seed foods as whole wheat, brown rice, rye, oats and corn, the following are excellent virility foods: millet, sesame seeds, sunflower seeds, pumpkin seeds, almonds and other raw nuts, beans, peas and peanuts.

6. MILK

Milk—of cow, goat, sheep, camel or mare, depending on the country and the continent—has been held in high repute as a potent virility food throughout man's history. The reason, whether determined in a laboratory or by actual use, is milk's protein content. The protein in milk, *casein, is the highest grade protein known to man.*

The biological value of protein is determined by its amino-acid content and proportions. All amino acids are important, but some of them can be synthetized in our system, some must be supplied with our food. Those that cannot be produced in our body and *must* come from the foods we eat, are called *essential amino acids.* There are ten of them. Foods that contain all ten are called complete protein foods. The right amounts of each amino acid in proportion to others is also of great importance. Milk protein is more "complete" than any other kind of protein—i.e. it has the highest biological value. In addition, milk protein is easily digested and more fully utilized than any other. Dr. James H. Leathem, of the Bureau of Biological Research at Rutgers University, said that sexual activity is stimulated by the hypophyseal hormone produced by the pituitary gland. This hormone is protein in nature and requires proteins in the diet for its production. The higher grade the protein, the higher the level of production of this sex-stimulant hormone.

Raw milk is also an excellent source of minerals, vitamins, trace elements and enzymes. Milk contains all the known vitamins, including the hard-to-get ones, D and B_{12}. Vitamin B_{12} is essential for sexual activity. It is found in large amounts in male seminal fluid and in the female uterus. It seems to be important for the healthy reproductive capacity of both men and women.

Liver is the best food source of vitamin B_{12}. Other sources are milk, cheese, eggs, fish and kelp. Some vegetables, grown on soils fertilized by manure, also contain certain amounts of vitamin B_{12}. But the scarcity of vitamin B_{12} in most foods of vegetable origin, emphasizes that the high-virility diet of vegetarians must include plenty of milk, milk products and possibly eggs.

Here is a special fortified milk cocktail to combat "bedroom fatigue" based on latest scientific findings as well as on ancient recipes:

PEP-UP COCKTAIL
(makes 2 glasses)

1½ glasses whole milk, preferably raw, unpasteurized.
2 tbsp. non-instant dry skim milk
2 egg yolks, raw
2 tbsp. raw, natural honey
1 tbsp. wheat germ oil
2 tbsp. fresh wheat germ
1 tbsp. sesame seeds
1 tbsp. pumpkin seeds
2 tsp. lecithin
1 tbsp. crushed ice

Place pumpkin seeds, sesame seeds, wheat germ, dry milk powder, and half of the milk in an electric blender (osterizer) and run for ½ to 1 minute, until seeds are well liquified. Add the rest of the milk, ice, egg yolks, honey, wheat germ oil, and lecithin and run again on high speed ten to fifteen seconds. Drink immediately. Sip slowly and enjoy its delicious, satisfying taste.

Make sure that all ingredients are fresh, especially wheat germ, wheat germ oil and sesame seeds. These foods turn rancid in a short time, and will taste somewhat bitter if not fresh. This formula will taste sweet and delicious if all the ingredients are fresh.

Pep-up Cocktail makes a perfect lunch for a busy, tired husband. Men with a weight problem can skip dinner now and then and replace it with a large glass of Pep-up Cocktail. This is a perfect, revitalizing drink for a tired wife, too.

While speaking of milk, we can't leave out yogurt. We have talked about the importance of high protein quality and of quick and thorough assimilation of protein. Milk protein is more completely and easily absorbed than any other, including that of meat. Well, yogurt is digested and utilized *twice as fast as ordinary milk!*

Yogurt is a "predigested" food, changed to this state by

bacterial action. In addition to being an instant source of complete proteins, yogurt is, like fresh milk, a storehouse of vitamins and minerals. It is also a delightfully refreshing food, perfect for a quick snack, dessert or as part of a bigger meal.

The fame and popularity of yogurt began with acclaim for its health-promoting and age-retarding properties. The Russian scientist Ilja Metchnikoff stated that putrefaction in the large intestine poisons the body and causes premature aging. He deduced that yogurt-eating Bulgarians and other Balkans live longer because the *lactobacillus bulgaricus,* the bacteria found in yogurt, destroys putrefactive bacteria in their intestines.

Yogurt consumption in the United States increased five hundred per cent in the last ten years. After being for decades a "health-faddist" food, sold only in health food stores and health bars, it is now in every supermarket. Latest figures shows annual sales of twenty-five million dollars.

Adelle Davis tells in her book LET'S GET WELL of a couple who had lost all interest in sex, but recaptured it on a diet she prescribed for their son; the diet specified increased milk intake and the addition of wheat germ and yeast. The couple told Miss Davis that her diet saved them from divorce.[3]

7. KELP

In Chapter 7 you read about the famous Chinese aphrodisiac, *Bird Nest Soup.* In the Orient, bird nest soup has been used for sexual vigor for thousands of years. The secret efficacy of the soup is in the seaweed plants and fish spawn from which the bird's nest is made. Seaweed—known

---

[3] Davis, Adelle, LET'S EAT RIGHT TO KEEP FIT, Harcourt, Brace & World, Inc., N.Y.

in the United States as kelp—is a wonder food of nature.

Kelp contains iodine, essential for the endocrine glands, especially the thyroid. Iodine deficiency can disrupt normal thyroid functions and cause diminished hormone production. Thyroid hormones are largely responsible for the sexual drive and stimulus. An underactive thyroid can diminish sexual vigor and libido. Kelp is the richest natural source of iodine It is also abundant in other vital minerals, such as magnesium, sodium, and potassium.

The importance of kelp as a part of human diet has been stressed by many researchers. Dr. Finn Batt, of Oslo, Norway, said that our soils are depleted in vital minerals and trace elements. He advised regular use of kelp to remedy trace-element deficiency. Finnish geologist, professor V. Auer, warned that man's health and reproductive capacity is in danger because food from depleted soils lacks the minerals and trace-elements which are vital for health. For thousands of years, minerals from tilled soils have been washed with the rains and rivers into the sea. These minerals are taken up by seaweed plants. Seaweed returns to man's diet what soils can no longer supply.

Seaweed as a food is not a modern fad, by any means. An ancient Chinese Book of Poetry, written in the eighth century B.C., tells of a housewife cooking seaweed for food. In China and Japan seaweed has always been a staple. In some parts of Japan seaweed provides one-fourth of the daily diet. Many western countries use seaweed extensively —for example, Ireland, Denmark, Scotland, Norway, Iceland, the Faroe Islands.

Seaweed has many varieties. In Ireland, the most popular kind is *dulse*, crisp and tender leaves called "sea lettuce." A seaweed that "looks like spinach and tastes like oysters," called *porphyra*, is eaten commonly in Scotland. In Japan, a large brown seaweed is used in soups, noodles, and served with rice. The same brown seaweed is used in the United States, as the source of kelp. Kelp is sold in health food stores in powder, granular or tablet form. It can be added to soups, breads, sauces, or sprinkled over potatoes and salads. Kelp has a strong salty taste and can be a salt substitute.

Kelp is an excellent source of minerals and trace elements. Dr. W.A.P. Black, of the British Nutrition Society, said that "seaweed contains all the elements that have so far been shown to play an important part in the physiological processes of man." [4] The vitamin C content of seaweed is very high—sometimes higher than in oranges. Seaweed has been the only source of vitamin C for many Eskimo groups. It also contains some vitamins B, A, E, K, and even B_{12}, which is seldom found in food of vegetable origin. In addition to potassium and chlorine, kelp contains trace minerals such as manganese, copper, silicon, boron, barium, lithium, strontium, zinc and vanadium. Dr. Black says that seaweed is an excellent source of minerals, because it grows in "an ideal environment." Sea water contains *all* the minerals needed for man's health. They are constantly renewed by nature, so there is no risk of depletion.

It would indeed, be wise to eat seaweed each day. The modern form of seaweed—kelp tablets—makes its use easier and cheaper, than cooking an expensive and elaborate *bird nest soup.*

8. FISH LIVER OIL

The importance of vitamin A for healthy function of your body, and particularly for the normal hormone production and the healthy mucous membranes and testicular tissue, was emphasized in detail in Chapter 10.

A recent national survey, reported by the U. S. Department of Agriculture, indicates that the vitamins most deficient in the American diet are A and C.

---

[4] *Proceedings of the Nutrition Society of England,* Vol. 12, 1953

Why this deficiency? The reason is that we don't eat the right kind of food. The best sources of vitamin A are fresh green, yellow or red vegetables and fruits. Carrots are the best vegetable source of carotene, a provitamin which is changed in the body into vitamin A. Fish, milk, butter and egg yolks are other good sources. But by far the best natural source of vitamin A is fish liver oil. Fish liver oils also contain large amounts of vitamin D, which is essential for the proper assimilation of minerals.

Since many people do not obtain enough vitamin A in their diet, they would be wise to use fish liver oils as a regular supplement. Once many people did not like the taste and smell—but today you can purchase fish liver oil *capsules* in drugstores or health food stores. They are easy to take and free from unwanted taste or odor.

When you buy fish liver oil, liquid or in capsules, make sure it is *pure fish liver oil with nothing added!* Most fish liver oil sold today contains added synthetic vitamins. Synthetic vitamins A and D may be harmful to your health in huge amounts, so avoid them unless prescribed by your doctor. Buy only plain fish liver oil, *not fortified.* Use according to the suggested dose on the label; two teaspoons a day is an approximate and moderate quantity.

9. LECITHIN

Lecithin, an organic phosphorized fat substance, is a chief constituent of brain and nerve tissues, and is also present in abundance in the endocrine glands, especially the gonads. Pituitary and pineal glands contain lecithin. The pineal gland is richer in lecithin than any other part of the body. Lecithin is also an essential component of semen and a sufficient supply is necessary for normal semen production.

Lecithin has another function about which much has been said in recent years. *Cholesterol* has lately become a villain, a mass murderer that kills people through plugged blood vessels and consequent heart attacks. Actually cholesterol is essential for good health. It is involved in many vital processes, including the production of adrenal and sex hormones, bile salts and formation of vitamin D. You need cholesterol. If it is not supplied by food, your body manufactures a certain amount. Why then all the fuss about avoiding cholesterol?

Not the cholesterol, but the body's ability to handle it, is the problem. To be utilized properly, cholesterol needs lecithin which is a natural emulsifier of fat. Lecithin prevents cholesterol from attaching in chunks to the walls of blood vessels and narrowing them so that blood movement is impeded. Lecithin, when given to persons with excessive cholesterol in the bloodstream, quickly emulsifies the cholesterol and carries it away. It seems that the problem is not too much cholesterol, but too little lecithin in the diet, that causes the hardening of arteries.

Is it possible to have a lecithin deficiency in your diet? Yes, it is very possible, because lecithin has been largely destroyed in food processing. Vegetable oils are excellent sources of lecithin, but hydrogenation of fats destroys lecithin. If you use hydrogenated shortenings, or eat restaurant food often, which is usually prepared with fat or fried in deep fat, you are ingesting great amounts of cholesterol *but no lecithin.* The lecithin, put in the fats by nature to act as an emulsifying agent for cholesterol, has been removed or destroyed in the hydrogenation process. This means that cholesterol will lump in your arteries and obstruct them.

For these reasons, lecithin is included in our ten special foods that can help to maintain your vigor. Fortunately, lecithin is now available in convenient and inexpensive form and is sold in every health food store.

The best way to prevent lecithin deficiency is to eat natural, unprocessed foods. Whole grains and seeds are rich sources of lecithin, especially soybeans and sesame seeds.

Eggs are especially rich in lecithin. Cold-pressed unprocessed vegetable oils are rich in lecithin, vitamin E and the essential fatty acids—all vital virility foods. In the process of hydrogenation, most lecithin, vitamin E and essential fatty acids have been destroyed. Considering the huge amounts of hydrogenated fats—shortenings and margarines—consumed in this country, is it any wonder that heart disease is our greatest killer and that even our children and teenagers suffer from arteriosclerosis in increasing numbers?

Here is what you can do to avoid the cholesterol problem and assure a plentiful supply of lecithin in your diet:

1. Avoid fat animal meat—the chief source of cholesterol.
2. Eat only unprocessed, natural whole-grain products.
3. Never use hydrogenated fats (shortenings, margarines) in any form.
4. Use cold-pressed, unprocessed vegetable oils liberally.
5. Take three teaspoons of granular lecithin (one with each meal) every day.

Commercial granulated or powdered lecithin is made from soybeans and is a rich source of choline and inositol, two important B-vitamins. There is evidence that deficiency of these two vitamins and of linoleic acid (essential fatty acid abundant in vegetable oils) is associated with coronary occlusion and coronary thrombosis, the major causes of death in the United States. Not only does hydrogenation destroy lecithin, but even refined vegetable oils lack it, because lecithin is discarded in the refining process. So be sure to buy unrefined cold-pressed vegetable oils. Health food stores sell them.

In addition to being an excellent help in preventing hardening of the arteries and feeding your brain, nerves, and sex glands, lecithin is beneficial in many other ways. It helps in the absorption of vitamin A and fats, it improves the utilization of vitamin E, which is so important for the healthy function of the reproductive system; it can lower the insulin requirement in diabetics, and has been used to treat psoriasis with excellent results.

10. EGGS

As you noted in Chapter 7, eggs have been a treasured aphrodisiac food throughout the ages. Eggs, milk, and honey are three foods most frequently credited with increasing sexual vigor and desire.

Eggs are one of the few foods used universally. In almost every culture, eggs have been looked upon as a symbol of fertility and used ceremonially, as Christians use them at Easter, to signify rebirth.

The folklore reputation of eggs as fertility and virility builders is solidly supported by modern nutritional research.

First, eggs are an abundant source of high quality protein. For the intricate workings of the endocrine and sex glands and for normal sex hormone production, the *quality* of protein is of great importance. As we have seen, milk provides the highest grade of protein for this purpose. *The egg protein is second only to milk protein in its biological value.* There are nutritionists who consider it the equal of milk. The quality of protein is determined by the correct quantity and proportion of the essential amino acids, the building blocks of protein. Egg proteins are extremely high in biological value by this standard of measure. One egg contains about six grams of high-quality protein.

Second, eggs are an excellent source of vitamins and minerals. All vitamins are well represented with the exception of vitamin C. Eggs are a particularly good source of vitamin A and all the B-vitamins. Even vitamin D is contained in eggs—and very few foods contain this vitamin. Eggs are rich in important minerals, especially in phosphorus and potassium. They are an abundant source of iron—1.1 milligram in each egg. In addition they contain copper which the body needs for utilization of iron. Iron deficiency is quite common in this country, especially among children and women.

Few foods available today have escaped processing or chemical tampering—eggs are one of them. The shell protects it from coming in direct contact with insecticides, preservatives and other toxic chemicals.

The darkness of the egg yolk supplies some indication of its mineral and vitamin content—the darker the yolk, the higher its nutritional value. The taste and nutritional value of eggs produced by farm hens is also superior to factory-produced eggs.

Egg yolks contain much cholesterol. For this reason some authorities advise cutting down on egg consumption, especially for those who have coronary problems. However, egg yolks also contain large amounts of lecithin, which is an emulsifier of cholesterol. It seems that the lecithin content in eggs is sufficient to prevent abnormal cholesterol metabolism. The real danger, from the cholesterol point of view, is in animal fats that contain huge amounts of cholesterol but no lecithin. Here is something to think about—Seventh-day Adventists abstain from meat eating for religious reasons. But they eat large quantities of eggs. Recent studies show that they have forty per cent less heart disease and hardening of the arteries than the overall American average.

One warning about eggs. Because the reputation of eggs is so widespread, some men consume many raw eggs daily. I knew a Swedish bachelor who consumed five or six raw eggs every day, claiming that they gave him phenomenal masculine power and endurance. Although I had no reason to doubt his testimony, I would not advise this many eggs for a prolonged regimen. Here is the reason. It has been shown in animal studies that raw egg white contains *avidin,* a substance that destroys (or binds) biotin, one of the B-vitamins produced in the intestines. There is, therefore, a danger that prolonged consumption of large amounts of raw egg white may result in severe biotin deficiency. *Avidin is destroyed in cooking.* For this reason, the egg white should be cooked, while egg yolk is the best eaten raw. The ideal way to eat eggs is to soft-boil them, so that the white will be cooked while the yolk remains raw. Another way is to separate whites from yolks, poach the white and use the yolk raw.

BRIEF SUMMARY OF CHAPTER 11

1. The basic premise of this book is that optimal nutrition can improve your general state of health, and that a high level of health is imperative for optimum sexual power.

2. In addition to the foods necessary for a high level of health, certain special food substances have a particularly beneficial effect on maintaining and enhancing our sexual vigor. These ten special foods are:

   1. Wheat germ
   2. Wheat germ oil
   3. Sesame seeds
   4. Honey
   5. Raw nuts and seeds
   6. Milk
   7. Kelp
   8. Fish liver oil
   9. Lecithin
   10. Eggs

3. These foods are *not* aphrodisiacs, but excellent sources of nutrients needed by the endocrine and sex glands for healthy functioning. They are not drugs or artificial stimulants, but natural and *hundred per cent harmless foods.*

CHAPTER 12

HOW TO PREVENT PREMATURE AGING

EVERY WOMAN EXPERIENCES "change of life," or menopause, most often between the ages of forty and fifty. Menopause means the end of the reproductive capacity. The ovaries cease releasing ova. Menstruation ends. This change may have a profound effect on a woman's personality and stability.

Is the change peculiar to women or do men have it too? Authorities seem to agree that a man's life has a comparable period. Men may not lose their reproductive power but they can have certain psychological symptoms during the critical age. This age can start as early as the late thirties, or as late as the end of fifties. Its duration can be anywhere between ten months and four years, according to such authorities as Kurt Mendel, Havelock Ellis and Kennet Walker. The period is characterized by sudden change in mood, unusual nervousness, anxiety, excessive sensitiveness, asocial tendencies, irritability, lack of confidence, etc.

Opinion is divided as to the real cause of these personality changes. Some think they are due to genital decay and slowed-down glandular activity. Others suggest that the symptoms are non-organic and caused by a man's realization that the dreams of youth are unfulfilled.

Whatever the cause or symptoms, one thing is definitely clear—man's fertility and his sex drive are not limited by age. A noted authority, Dr. Flanders Dunbar, made a study of American centenarians. He questioned twenty per cent of all individuals over ninety-nine. When asked at what age each had lost interest in sex, most said they had not reached it. Many of these men still retained their potency. Some remarried after passing the century mark. This has also been reported from Hunza, "the healthiest nation in the world," where men have been known to father children after reaching the age of ninety or one hundred, as told by R. Taylor in his book HUNZA HEALTH SECRETS.[1]

LIFE-LONG POTENCY IS MAN'S BIRTHRIGHT

A certain decline in male sexual desires and ability is normal as the years advance. Man's sex glands reach a peak at twenty or twenty-two. Hormone and sperm production diminish as man grows older—*but very slowly.*

Under favorable conditions, lifelong sexuality is man's birthright. Although a man in his sixties cannot be as active as in his twenties, at no physiological age does man's sexual ability come to a suddent halt.

Why are so many men impotent? The answer is not that they are old, but that they are *insufficiently healthy.* Impotence is a symptom common to many forms of ill health. The body tries to protect itself from overexertion by causing temporary impotence. Sexuality is the result of

[1] Taylor, R., HUNZA HEALTH SECRETS, Prentice-Hall, Inc., Inglewood Cliffs, N.J. 1964

an extra, unused energy. When all available energy is needed to fight for life, none is left for sex.

While in younger men most impotence is caused by non-organic, psychic factors, in older men the physiological causes are common. Kinsey studies indicated that decline in sexual activity of the older male is often the result of general decline in his physiological capacity.

OTHER FACTORS AFFECTING MAN'S VIRILITY AFTER 40

Often, the decline of sexual virility in middle-aged man is due to a lack of motivation. As Dr. Jessie Bernard suggests, too little stimulation may remain in a relationship which has become routinized. Some wives destroy a husband's libido by derision—not to mention what they do to him in the kitchen.

A man's declined sexual interest is also due to lack of sufficient exercise and resultant fat and flab. Regular walking or jogging can help keep the body fit—but too many will not bother.

Excessive use of drugs is another common reason for declined virility. Many common medicines interfere with sexual response, especially the sedatives and tranquilizers. Any drug which depresses the central nervous system can cause impotence in men.[2]

Smoking and drinking are definitely detrimental. According to Dr. A. P. Runciman, of the Reproductive Biology Research Foundation in St. Louis, excessive use of alcohol can be blamed more than anything else for sexual impotence in males over fifty.

Devitalized nutrition is always a factor, as is the growing toxicity of our environment.

---

[2] Rubin, Isadore, Ph.D., SEXUAL LIFE AFTER SIXTY, Basic Books, Inc., Publishers, N.Y., 1965

DOES OBESITY DIMINISH SEXUAL LIBIDO?

Naturally! Here is an illustration. Take two men of the same age, the same stature, in similar circumstances and doing the same kind of work, both weighing one hundred fifty pounds. Let one of the men carry a forty-pound sand bag on his back all day, from the time he gets out of bed until he returns to it. Which of these men will have more energy left for sexual interest?

Yet this is exactly what a man, forty pounds overweight is doing every day! Keep in mind that sexual desire is sparked by *excess* energy. An overweight man is so exhausted by carrying his own fat all day long that he has no energy left for amorous interests. A fat man may be jolly, but he is certainly never a great lover. Not only does he look older than his age, but he feels older too. With fork and knife he is aging himself prematurely, also sexually speaking. Dr. Belham said, "Leanness, long life and virility all go together".[3]

Obesity is one of the worst enemies of virility. And obesity is almost always caused by overeating. Why do people overeat? Largely because they eat devitalized foods which have been robbed of vital nutrients. When we eat refined, devitalized foods, nutrients are missing which are needed to convert food into energy. Thus, although we eat a lot, we still feel hungry and eat more. If calories are not converted into energy, they are stored in the body as fat.

FEMALE AND MALE MENOPAUSE MAY BE FAVORABLY AFFECTED BY PROPER NUTRITION

The secret of staying young and virile is basically the secret of staying healthy.

---

[3] Belham, George, THE VIRILITY DIET, Dell Publishing Co., Inc., N.Y. 1968 Copyright (c) 1965 by George Belham

Menopause may start for some women in the late thirties. In other cases women continue to menstruate in the early fifties. The reason for the difference is largely hormonal. A devitalized nutrition can result in starved endocrine and sexual glands, causing a woman to age prematurely. Mrs. L., of whom I spoke in Chapter 4, had all the signs of a premature menopause when she was thirty-five. When she started to feed her glands properly, all symptoms of premature menopause and premature aging disappeared as if by magic. After a couple of years on a revitalizing diet, her friends could hardly recognize her. She looked ten years younger and had regained all her former interest and self-confidence.

A good friend of mine, George M., was a few years past forty when one day he said to me, "I don't know what's the matter with me . . . I may be getting old. At what age is a man supposed to quit, anyway?" He tried to laugh, but his expression and voice revealed a serious concern for his waning masculine power. "Do you think some pills of yours may help?" he continued.

"I don't think pills alone will do the trick," I said. "What you need, old chap, is a thorough overhaul of your mistreated and malnourished body. Your starved glands are slowing down their hormone production because you have neglected to feed them properly. You wouldn't think of running your car on low-grade gas or inferior oil, but when it comes to your own body you kick it around like junk. How can you expect to run in high-gear and perform efficiently when you don't have the proper fuel?"

I had warned George for years of the inevitable consequences of his health-destroying living and eating habits. But most people are not interested in health until it starts to elude them. Now George was willing to listen, willing to try anything to regain his withering masculinity.

I outlined a program for him. I told him it would be long-term. Years of abuse had dragged him down—and it would take him months, perhaps years, to regain health and recapture his dwindling potency. He was to stop smoking and drinking. (He did not stop completely, but cut down drastically on both.) He was to take regular exercise, daily walking and jogging, and lose twenty pounds. He had to change his eating habits; avoiding white sugar, white flour and everything made from them, while learning to like fresh fruits and vegetables, milk and yogurt, nuts, seeds and whole grain products. In addition, I advised him to use the special foods described in Chapters 9 and 11 of this book.

I learned long ago not to advise reasonably healthy people to take care of their health—they are not sufficiently interested or alarmed to make the effort of application. Many have tried half-heartedly to change their living and eating habits, but usually gave up after a few days or weeks. One of the most pathetic comments I have heard, among a great number of excuses, is, "I'd rather live ten years less, but eat what I like." People fail to realize that the alternative is not ten years more or less, but a choice between vibrant health and a state of constant chronic fatigue.

George M. knew that he had to choose between these two alternatives. He was ready for what turned out to be, in his own words, uttered three years later, the most important decision of his life.

Miraculous transformation is a cliché expression, but I cannot find better words to describe what happened to George in a few short months. His wife reported that George had changed from a sullen, grumpy individual to a happy and cheerful one. His office employees were pleasantly surprised to have their boss become less critical, less demanding, more tolerant. His children were delighted with their father's interests in their school work and his willingness to play with them. His outbursts of temper ceased. Suddenly George started to sing in his shower again, as he had done during his first years of marriage. I have followed George on many jogging trips. I saw him shed pound after pound from his heavy frame. He also reported a new surge of sexual interest. And at a party a few months later, his wife whispered to me, "Thanks for what you did for George. It's like having a second honeymoon."

Actually no miracle was involved in George's transformation. Hundreds of other men have responded to improved nutrition and corrected living habits in a similar way. The causes of Mr. M.'s lowered sexual vigor were many—overweight, heavy smoking and drinking, devitalized nutrition, constant preoccupation with business problems and worries. But most of these underlying causes affected his masculine power through the endocrine glands. Alcohol and tobacco have, of course, a direct potency-destroying effect. Devitalized nutrition starved his gonads and other vital glands and depleted their supply of hormones. The lack of male sex hormone testosterone brought about unpleasant psychological changes in his character and also contributed to the dwindling of his potency.

By cutting down on smoking and drinking (by the way, after one year of the revitalizing program, he stopped smoking completely) and by strictly adhering to the high-virility diet (with all the special vitamins and food supplements) his glandular activity was soon restored, the functions of his vital organs and glands revitalized, the nerve and muscle strength reestablished. He acquired emotional stability and more physical strength. Thus, premature climacteric symptoms and early sexual senility were prevented.

The modern science of gerontology is busily engaged in research on the aging process. The final and conclusive results are not available as yet, but one major factor has been clearly pointed out—nutrition.

Dr. Henry C. Sherman of Columbia University, one of the greatest authorities on nutrition, has said that human life can be extended and youthfulness preserved by the right selection of foods. Devitalized nutrition causes premature aging of tissues and all vital organs. Dr. Tom Spies has said that we can make old age wait by correcting nutritional deficiencies.

HOW TO PREVENT SEXUAL SENILITY WITH IMPROVED NUTRITION

Here are, in summary, vital points to remember:

1. Life-long potency is every man's birthright.
2. Man's libido, after he has reached middle age, is more often than not adversely affected by several organic and physiological causes, such as smoking and drinking, obesity, various degrees of ill health, excessive use of drugs. These libido-destroying factors must be checked and corrected before the full benefits of improved nutrition can be realized.
3. Proper nutrition stands as a fortress against premature aging generally and against premature sexual senility in particular.

In a nutshell, for preserving continuing good health and maintaining sexual ability follow these rules:

- Do not smoke or drink. Smoking and drinking can cause impotence.
- Keep slim. Leanness, long life, and virility go hand in hand.
- Avoid undue emotional stresses and worries: have a happy, positive outlook on life.
- Keep fit by regular exercise. Walking is the best form of exercise for older people.
- Check with your doctor for possible pathological reasons for ill health and correct all the diseased conditions. Impotence is a common symptom of many diseases.
- Avoid drugs. Many common drugs can lower your virility.
- See that your diet is health and virility-building, not virility-destroying. Part Two of this book will teach you the basic rules of health and virility-building nutrition.

CHAPTER 13

CAN PROSTATE PROBLEMS BE PREVENTED BY NUTRITIONAL MEANS?

PROSTATE TROUBLES HAVE reached epidemic proportions. Reliable medical estimates are that four out of five men will have prostate trouble in one form or another. The most common disorder is prostate enlargement, which is characterized by excessive tissue growth inside the gland and around it. The enlargement causes obstruction of the bladder, which may lead to painful infections and inflammations.

The prostate is a sex gland, about the size of a chestnut, which encircles the neck of the urethra. The gland secretes an alkaline fluid that is mixed with semen. Although it is possible to have satisfactory sexual relations and even successful impregnation after the surgical removal of the prostate gland, prostate disorders and the pathological developments connected with them may result in impaired fertility and an inability to have sexual intercourse.

WHAT CAUSES PROSTATE DISORDERS

The causes of prostate disorders are many. Some cases of acute inflammation of the prostate are a result of neglected gonorrhea. In other cases a tuberculous infection may occur, usually as a result of tuberculosis in the kidneys or other genito-urinary organs.

Prostate disorders may be connected with sexual activity. During excitement the sexual apparatus becomes engorged with blood. This is true not only of the penis, where blood engorgement makes erection possible, but also of all accessory sexual organs, including the prostate gland. After normal heterosexual intercourse which culminates in orgasm, this blood engorgement subsides rapidly and all sexual organs return to a relaxed state. But certain sexual practices, although achieving a high degree of excitation, do not lead to quick conclusion and gratification. Prolonged excitation with suppressed ejaculation constitutes a definite abuse of the sexual glands, especially of the prostate gland. Here are some of the harmful sexual practices that may lead to prostate disorders: [1]

- The practice of advanced petting which leads to a high degree of sexual excitation and engorgement without a natural conclusion.
- The practice of withdrawal or incomplete sexual act without orgasm.
- Excessive deliberate prolongation of the sexual act, during which the approaching ejaculation is suppressed.
- Overindulgence or undue abstinence from sexual gratification.

CAN PROSTATE DISORDERS BE PREVENTED?

When prostate trouble has gone too far, when there is an infectious condition and serious difficulty in urinating,

[1] Kenyon, Herbert R., M.D., THE PROSTATE GLAND, Random House, N.Y., 1950

the only sensible course is to seek medical help. Self-diagnosis and self-medication are certainly not advisable in cases of advanced prostate disorder.

But if you are not yet troubled with serious prostate distress you will be interested in preventive techniques and good health habits.

An early study of the relation between nutrition and prostate disorders involves unsaturated fatty acids, or vitamin F and lecithin. Researchers in Los Angeles treated nineteen patients with unsaturated fatty acids. No other treament was given and the results were remarkable. All cases showed a lessening of residual urine. Thirteen out of nineteen patients could stop getting up at night. In all cases the size of the prostate gland was rapidly reduced.[2] Unsaturated fatty acids are plentiful in cold-pressed vegetable oils and in all unrefined seeds and whole grains.

The other natural substance used successfully for the treatment of prostate disorders is pollen. Dr. Ask-Upmark, Uppsala, Sweden, reported a case of a man who suffered from acute prostate inflammation (prostatovesiculitis) for five years and was treated unsuccessfully with conventional drugs, including antibiotics. After treatment with *cernilton,* a pollen preparation, his prostate problems completely disappeared. A very extensive study was made a few years later by three Swedish researchers, Dr. Gösta Leander, Professor Gösta Jonsson, and Professor H. Palmstierna at the urological clinic of the University of Lund. They reported that strictly controlled tests on one hundred seventy-nine cases of chronic prostate inflammation showed that *cernilton,* in combination with conventional treatments, gave better results than the conventional therapy alone.[3]

---

[2] Pamphlet published by Lee Foundation for Nutritional Research, 2023 W. Wisconsin Ave., Milwaukee, Wisc. (Nov. 1941)

[3] Essén, Lars-Erik, M.D., POLLEN SOM LÄKEMEDEL, Vita Nova Förlag, Mölle, Sweden

By 1965 their studies included over eleven hundred cases, with the same positive results.

Pollen is now collected with special machines constructed for the purpose. Pollen and pollen preparations are sold in drugstores and health food stores in European countries, and also in health food stores in the United States. What part of pollen is active in prostate disorder is not known, but Dr. Ask-Upmark thinks that the small amounts of plant hormone in pollen may be responsible.[3]

ZINC AND PROSTATE DISORDERS

Scientists are convinced that the dietary deficiency of zinc and/or ineffective zinc absorption, are closely related to the deterioration of the prostate gland.

Dr. W. Devrient, of Germany, was the first scientist to discover that pumpkin seeds preserve the health of the prostate gland. He also suggested that pumpkin seeds are a powerful source of the virility-and potency-building materials.[4] In countries where pumpkin seeds are eaten regularly and in great quantity, there is virtually no prostate trouble. Pumpkin seeds are rich in zinc.

Dr. André Voisin, famous French nutritionist, refers in his book SOIL, GRASS AND CANCER, to research done at the Winnipeg hospital in Canada. The Winnipeg research clearly showed that even a mild deficiency of zinc in the diet causes a noticeable enlargement of the prostate gland. The same study showed that a serious deficiency of zinc may lead to cancer in the prostate.[5]

Adelle Davis, the famous American nutritionist, reported that vitamin C is an effective agent in correcting prostate

---

[4] Rodale, J. I., and staff, THE COMPLETE BOOK ON FOOD AND NUTRITION, Rodale Books, Inc., Emmaus, Penna., 1961

[5] Voisin, André, SOIL, GRASS AND CANCER, Philosophical Press

infections. She gave large amounts of vitamin C to four men with prostate infections with excellent results.[6] The excessive use of alcohol[7] and excessive smoking[8] are also reported as predisposing causative factors in prostate disorders. Dr. E. Löffelman, of Tubingen, Germany, names coffee and irritating spices as predisposing causes.[9]

The late Dr. Benjamin F. Sieve, of Boston, studied hundreds of prostate patients and found that most of them were in a low nutritional state. His nutritional treatments saved seventy per cent of the patients from surgery.[10] He emphasized that his treatments were purely preventive. Dr. Sieves' prescription was almost totally nutritional, except for the prostate massage given once a week. He advised a well-balanced diet plus all the known vitamins; A, B, C, D and E. In addition to large oral doses he also gave vitamin injections as well as a chlorophyl substance made from alfalfa, buckwheat and soybean.

SEVEN-POINT PROGRAM FOR PREVENTION OF PROSTATE DISORDERS

In summary, here is a seven-point program aimed at prevention of prostate disorders.

1. *Moderation* in sexual activity is of utmost importance. Avoid overindulgence, which can overstrain the prostate gland; avoid also undue abstinence especially after decades of regular sexual activity. Do not suppress the sexual urge.

---

[6] Davis, Adelle, LET'S GET WELL, Harcourt, Brace & World, Inc., N.Y., 1965

[7] Willy, A., et al., THE ILLUSTRATED ENCYCLOPEDIA OF SEX, Cadillac Publishing Co., Inc., N.Y.

[8] Devrient, W., Androgen-Hormonal Curative Influence of a Neglected Plant, Quoted in *Prevention,* September, 1959

[9] Löffelman, E., "When We Get Older", REFORMKURIREN, No. 11, September, 1965, Sweden

[10] *American Journal of Digestive Disorders,* December, 1951

Healthy men can and should enjoy sex as long as they live.

2. Avoid sexual excitation without a natural conclusion in the form of ejaculation, or orgasm. Such habits as petting, withdrawal, and unduly prolonged intercourse, are harmful for the prostate gland. They result in a prolonged engorgement (accumulation of blood) and suppressed or incomplete ejaculation which may lead to functional and even structural damage of the prostate gland.

3. Avoid excessive smoking and drinking—both are considered contributing causes of prostatitis predispostion.

4. See that your general health status is high. Optimum health is imperative for healthy organs and glands.

5. Exercise! Walking is the best possible form of exercise for keeping the prostate in good shape. One or two hours a day is not too much.

6. Deficiencies in zinc and vitamin F have been named as possible causes of prostate disorders. Inclusion of these nutrients in the diet has brought great improvement in prostate conditions. Empirical evidence shows that where people eat unrefined, natural foods rich in zinc and fatty acids, they are virtually free from prostate troubles. Dr. E. Loffelman recommends the following preventive dietary program for men over forty:

- Plenty of fresh vegetables and fruits for vitamins and minerals.
- Elimination of strong spices.
- Moderation in coffee and alcohol drinking.
- Fresh vitamin-rich vegetable and fruit juices to supplement the basic diet.

The best health-building diet—both for general health and for the health of the reproductive system, is outlined in Chapters 9, 10, and 11 of this book.

7. Supplement your diet with the following foods for the health of the prostate gland:

- Raw pumpkin and sunflower seeds for zinc and other valuable nutrients. These delicious seeds can be chewed as they are or powdered in an electric grinder to be mixed with milk or juice, or sprinkled over salads and cereals.

- Cold-pressed vegetable oils such as soybean oil, safflower oil, sunflower oil, corn oil, for unsaturated fatty acids, lecithin and vitamin E.
- Lecithin, one to two tablespoons daily, in granular, powder or liquid form.
- Rose hip tablets or other rich sources of vitamin C. Preventive dose: 200 to 300 milligrams daily. In case of prostate inflammation, take large doses of several thousand milligrams a day. Vitamin C is completely harmless even in large doses.
- Brewer's yeast, one to three tablespoons (or equivalent in tablets) a day for vitamins of the B-complex and for excellent proteins.
- Fish liver oil for vitamins A and D. Follow instructions on the bottle.
- Wheat germ oil for vitamin E and unsaturated fatty acids.

CHAPTER 14

HOW SEX AFFECTS YOUR HEART

HEART DISEASE IS the number one killer of our time. More people die from heart attacks than from all other causes combined. In the United States alone over 20 million people are afflicted with heart disease and arteriosclerosis. The International Conference on Thrombosis reports that more than one and a half million Americans will suffer heart attacks and strokes in 1970.[1] Statistics show that heart disease kills not only middle-aged and old people, but also young men and women. According to recent tests, seventy per cent of our youth between twenty and twenty-five suffer from various degrees of arteriosclerosis—the condition which often leads to heart failure.[2] However, the people most vulnerable to heart attacks are not old or young, but men and women in the prime of life. After years of hard work and study, at the crest of their professional or business careers, just when they should be harvesting the

[1] Report at *The International Conference on Thrombosis,* November 29, 1967

[2] Evers, Joseph, M.D., THE CHANGED ASPECTS OF DISEASES

fruits of their labor, men succumb to heart attack in increasing numbers.

HEART DISEASE AND SEX

Hundreds of books have been published in recent years on heart disease, its causes and prevention. Scientific discourses, as well as popular paperbacks, treat the problem of heart disease from every possible angle, expect one—*sex*. Every aspect of heart disease is discussed in detail. All possible causes and forms of stress are ventilated—faulty diet, lack of exercise, cholesterol, emotional stress, smoking. But most doctors and researchers, abiding by the unwritten law that considers sex a "forbidden" subject, ignore or avoid the issue of sex in relation to heart disease. Only recently, some reports shed light on this vital question.

Two scientists from the Reproductive Biology Research Foundation in St. Louis, Missouri, William H. Masters, M.D., and Virginia Johnson, have conducted extensive studies on volunteers and reported the results in a book called HUMAN SEXUAL RESPONSE.[3] A few other scientific studies have been made in this field, notably one made in Germany by Doctors Klumbies and Kleinsorge, and another by Dr. R. G. Bartlett, Jr. in the United States.[4] The German study was limited to the effect of masturbation and the resultant orgasm on the circulatory system and the heart. Dr. Bartlett's study concerned married couples engaged in sexual intercourse.

All these studies reported similiar results: sexual intercourse has a profound effect on blood pressure, heartbeat

---

[3] Masters, W. H., and Johnson, V. E., HUMAN SEXUAL RESPONSE, Little, Brown & Co., Boston, 1966

[4] Bartlett, R. G., Jr., Physiologic Responses During Coitus, *Journal of Applied Physiology*, November, 1956

and the breathing rate. In the Bartlett study, the heartbeat rate reached 170 beats per minute and the breathing rate, both husbands' and wives', rose close to 70 breaths per minute at the time of orgasm. In the Master and Johnson studies, men and women showed heartbeat rates up to 180 or even higher during orgasm. Blood pressure elevations reached 80 mm. for systolic and 50 mm. for diastolic pressure over the normal. In the German experiments, the systolic blood pressure leaped to nearly 250 mm. at orgasm.

These studies show that sexual intercourse is an extremely strenuous activity and puts a great demand on the various vital organs, especially the heart. The logical questions are: Is sexual intercourse dangerous for persons with a record of cardiac incident? Can frequent sex weaken a healthy heart?

"DEATH ON TOP OF TUMMY"

French call it *la mort d'amour;* our doctors usually report on the death certificate "died in sleep"; but the Japanese have a more descriptive phrase to refer to the so-called coition death, or death while making love—in literal translation it means "death on top of tummy." [5] Both ancient and modern literature describe men dying during a sexual act. Death from heart attack during coitus is not reported as such in the death certificates or obituary columns in our country.

Can love kill, as was recently suggested in "Love Can Kill" in an Esquire article?

In an excellent book, SEX AND YOUR HEART,[6]

---

[5] Ueno, Masahiko, M.D., "The So-called Coition Death", *Japanese Journal of Legal Medicine,* September, 1963

[6] Brenton, Myron, SEX AND YOUR HEART, Coward-McCann, Inc., New York, 1968

Myron Brenton treats the relation between sex activity and the heart. His conclusions are that patients with heart disease should exercise moderation. For healthy individuals, sexual intercourse, of course, causes no more physical damage than any other form of strenuous exercise. On the contrary, it is definitely beneficial to the heart and circulatory system, as well as the physique generally. For someone with a weak heart or advanced coronary atheroselerosis, sexual intercourse can be dangerous.

Documented cases of death during coitus are not many, but nevertheless not rare enough to ignore. Dr. M. Ueno reported that of 5,559 cases he investigated 34 sudden deaths were definitely related to sexual activity. Dr. George Trimble also reported several cases of heart attack during coitus.[7] Similar reports have been published in the Journal of the American Medical Association and the Journal of Applied Physiology. The scarcity of information in this area is often caused by reluctance of those involved to give the attending physician the correct information.

SHOULD AN INDIVIDUAL WITH HEART DISEASE ENGAGE IN SEXUAL ACTIVITY?

Certainly! Abstinence from sex can be as damaging to the heart as overindulgence. Sexual intercourse is a normal biological process. Lack of sexual expression can cause emotional and physical stress. The frustrations and tensions caused by lack of sexual gratification can be as bad for the heart as sexual overindulgence.

Most heart patients can and should enjoy sexual relations, although with caution and moderation. Certain habits and techniques will reduce the excitement connected with sex-

---

[7] Trimble, G. X., *Journal of The American Medical Association,* June 7, 1965

ual intercourse and keep physical and emotional stress to the minimum.

Sex-related heart attacks may occur under circumstances of heightened excitement, such as occasional affairs with a new partner. Dr. Masahiko Ueno reported that most deaths related to sexual activity occured under circumstances other than normal martial relations, an overwhelming majority in hotels, with the men much older than their partners. This seems to indicate that illicit sex will heighten stress and place an extra burden upon the heart. Sex within marriage, after many years of experience, usually provides a relaxed atmosphere and is less strenuous for the heart.

HEART, SEX, AND NUTRITION

The risk of a heart attack during coitus is considerably diminished for a heart in optimum condition. As we have seen, the heartbeat during orgasm may leap to an astonishing three beats per second. The muscles of your heart need fresh oxygen for every beat. Rapid breathing, of course, indicates that your heart needs more oxygen for its accelerated activity. This is where *vitamin E*—a miracle heart saver—enters the picture.

YOUR HEART AND VITAMIN E

Vitamin E has three marvelous properties which assist good heart and artery function:

1. Vitamin E preserves oxygen in the blood and markedly reduces the need for intake of oxygen.
2. Vitamin E is a powerful anti-coagulant and can prevent death through thrombosis or blood clot.
3. Vitamin E is a dilator of blood vessels. It can im-

prove circulation and increase the flow of blood to the heart when an extra supply is needed.

Evan S. Shute, M.D., of the Shute Foundation in Canada, the foremost authority on the use of vitamin E in the treatment of heart disease, says, "Vitamin E is the most valuable ally the cardiologist has yet found . . . It is the key both to the prevention and treatment of all those conditions in which a lack of blood supply due to thickened or blocked blood vessels or a lack of oxygen is a factor or the whole story of the disease".[8]

Whether it be for an already damaged heart or as a safety measure to protect your heart and prevent a heart attack, vitamin E is an indispensable aid. Heart disease may have many contributing causes, such as nutritional deficiencies, lack of exercise, obesity, smoking or emotional stress. But the way all these factors affect the heart is the same—they cause an oxygen deficiency in the heart muscle, which, in severe cases, results in heart attack. The need for oxygen in your heart can be doubled or tripled during sexual intercourse. Vitamin E will reduce the need for oxygen by as much as forty-three per cent. Its powerful anti-coagulant and blood-vessel-dilating action can prevent heart attack and, consequently, save your life.

Foods rich in vitamin E are wheat germ, wheat germ oil, whole grains and whole grain products, raw nuts and seeds, cold pressed vegetable oils. Processed breakfast cereals and white bread are poor sources of vitamin E. Vitamin E also can be bought in capsule form from a drugstore or health food store. Most doctors recommend 300 International Units per day as a preventive measure, and up to 600 a day for heart cases. If you have heart disease, consult your doctor for a suitable dosage.

---

[8] ENCYCLOPEDIA FOR HEALTHFUL LIVING, Rodale Books, Inc., Emmaus, Penna., 1960

YOUR HEART AND VITAMIN C

Another vitamin involved in the health of your heart is *vitamin C.* Clinical studies reveal that 81 per cent of coronary patients have a subnormal level of vitamin C in the blood.[9] Dr. W.J. McCormick says that deficiency of vitamin C is one cause of coronary thrombosis.[10] This deficiency can cause ruptures in the blood vessel walls and lead to heart attack. Vitamin C strengthens the walls of blood vessels and capillaries, as well as all the connective tissues and muscles of the body. Russian scientists have found that vitamin C can reduce the amount in cholesterol in the blood. Up to fifty per cent decline in cholesterol was noticed twenty-four hours after giving a patient vitamin C.[11] These few samples should be sufficient to impress upon you that your diet should contain plenty of vitamin C.

Foods rich in vitamin C are fresh fruits and vegetables. Rose hips and acerola cherries are the best natural sources of vitamin C. You can buy vitamin C in tablet form, of course, in your drug or health food store. Doses of one thousand milligrams or more a day are recommended in cases where there is a history of heart failure.

OTHER NUTRITIONAL FACTORS

Accumulated research tends to show that *B-vitamins* also play an important role in the prevention and treatment of heart disease. *Thiamine* (B_1) deficiency has been found to

---

[9] *Canadian Medical Association Journal,* Vol. 44, 114, 1941

[10] McCormick, W. J., M.D., Coronary Thrombosis, *Clinical Medicine,* Vol. 4:7, 1957

[11] Miasnikov, I. A., *Terapevtichevskij Arkhiv,* Vol. 28, 1956

impair the function of the heart,[12] also *niacin, pyridoxine* and *choline*—all vitamins of the B complex—have both prophylactic and therapeutic value in heart disease.

Among other nutritional factors, the following minerals and trace elements have been connected with heart disease: calcium, magnesium, vanadium, zinc and potassium. The British Medical Journal reports that a significant decrease in heart disease mortality could be achieved by an increased dietary intake of *calcium*. Recent studies in Switzerland link heart disease with *magnesium* deficiency.[13]

Linolenic acid, present in flaxseed oil and soybean oil, and *lecithin,* from soybeans, have heart-attack preventive properties. Dr. Paul A. Owren, a Norwegian medical researcher, has demonstrated that one tablespoon of purified linseed (flaxseed) oil a day can prevent heart attacks caused by blood clots. Lecithin also prevents clot formation and thus diminishes risk of an attack.

As you can see, you can do much to minimize the stress on your heart with nutrition.

NUTRITIONAL PROGRAM FOR STRONGER HEART

To prevent a potential heart attack and to meet increased stress caused by sexual activity, here is an eight-point program of do's and don'ts:

1. See that your diet contains vital elements needed to keep your body and your heart in perfect health. See Chapter 9 for the complete description of a balanced diet for optimum health.

2. Supplement your diet with vitamins, minerals,

---

[12] Eddy, Walter H., Ph.D. and Dalldorf, Gilbert, M.D., THE AVITAMINOSES, Williams & Wilkins Company

[13] Goldsmith, Naomi F., et al., *Archives of Environmental Health,* May, 1966

vegetable oils and lecithin as suggested in this chapter. Consult your doctor or nutritionist for proper dosage.

3. Avoid excessive amount of animal protein and animal fats. A recent study shows that Seventh-Day Adventists, who do not eat meat, have 40 per cent less blood vessel and heart disease compared with American average.

4. Avoid white sugar, white flour, soft drinks, cakes and pies, ice cream and other sweets. Dr. John Yudkin of London University suggests that excessive consumption of white sugar and other refined carbohydrates is a *prime cause of heart disease*. Dr. B.P. Sandler has demonstrated that high intake of refined carbohydrate causes abnormal fluctuations in blood sugar levels and may lead to oxygen deficiency in the heart.[14]

5. Do not overeat. Keep slim. The Metropolitan Life Insurance Company tells us that the death rate from heart disease is fifty per cent higher among the overweight. Especially avoid heavy eating before sexual intercourse. The digestive process requires a great amount of blood—and so does sexual activity. Your heart may not be able to meet the demand for this double duty.

6. Avoid alcohol. Alcohol is a cardiac stimulant and puts an extra strain on the heart. It also loosens inhibitions, impairs judgment and may lead a person with a weak heart to more strenuous sexual effort than he can stand.

7. Avoid coffee, tea and cola drinks. They stimulate the heart and increase the blood sugar level *temporarily*, after which it drops to dangerous levels, possibly causing an oxygen deficiency in heart muscle tissues. This could be fatal during coitus.

8. Finally, avoid emotional tensions, anxieties, and fears, especially connected with sex. Don't try to prove anything to yourself or your partner. Do not engage in sex while fatigued or after a meal. Many older people, especially heart

---

[14] Sandler, B. P., M.D., How to Prevent Heart Attacks, *Lee Foundation for Nutritional Research,* Milwaukee, Wisc.

cases, find that the best time for coitus is in the morning, after a night of rest and in a relaxed state of mind.

BRIEF SUMMARY OF THIS CHAPTER

1. Heart disease is the number one killer of Americans, the most dreadful epidemic of modern times.
2. Sexual intercourse has a profound effect on the heart. It increases the heartbeat, elevates the blood pressure and raises the breathing rate.
3. Although deaths from heart attack caused by coitus are rare, they do occur. A person who has a weak heart, or a history of coronary occulusions, should exercise moderation in relation to sex.
4. Abstinence from sex is not advocated, because it can cause emotional stress and frustrations which may affect the heart as adversely as overindulgence. Moderation and sex of a less intensive kind is recommended by doctors.
5. Demands made on the heart by sexual activity can be minimized by proper diet. Vitamins E, B, and C, the minerals calcium and magnesium, lecithin and vegetable oils have a strengthening effect on the heart and can be helpful in preventing attacks. The ultimate cause of heart attack is oxygen deficiency in the muscle tissues of the organ. Vitamin E reduces the need for oxygen. Vitamin E is a powerful heart-saver.
6. An-eight point program of protecting your heart with nutrition and other means, while enjoying a normal marital life.

CHAPTER 15

"IF HE KISSED YOU ONCE . . ."

NUMEROUS FACTORS AND problems, some major, some absurdly small, may interfere with the full enjoyment of a normal sexual union. The major problems are, of course, male impotence and female frigidity. Male impotence makes normal sexual intercourse almost impossible. Female frigidity not only prevents a woman from achieving a fulfilling orgasm, but also limits man's enjoyment of the sexual act.

But even in the case of a perfectly normal couple, when the man is virile and woman is warm and responsive, many seemingly insignificant things may spoil the full enjoyment of sex. Any kind or degree of ill health interferes with normal sex life in one way or another. Irritability, nagging, arguments, headache, chronic fatigue—all these can kill desire. A man's sustained erection and a woman's willing responsiveness can be nipped in the bud by such seemingly minor things as a sarcastic remark, a word of criticism, untidy or dirty clothing, unpleasant body odor—or halitosis. The problem of bad breath seems to increase with age, because of gradually deteriorating health, constipation, bad mouth hygiene or poorly cleaned dentures.

Mouthwash and breath-mint manufacturers have played

up the theme of halitosis and created a multi-million-dollar industry.

"If he kissed you once—will he kiss you again?" In dramatized television commercials bad breath has been blamed for complete failure in business and love. As a result, almost everyone in the United States now uses some kind of mouthwash or breath-candy.

What is the truth about halitosis and the mouthwashes? Do most of us really have bad breath? Does mouthwash remove it? What causes bad breath and how can it be prevented or eliminated?

Because bad breath, when it really does exist, can cause serious friction and be an irritating factor in achieving an enjoyable sexual relation, we should try to find true answers to these questions.

HALITOSIS ALMOST NONEXISTENT

How prevalent is bad breath? Mouthwash manufacturers imply that most of us are afflicted with halitosis. It makes one wonder how billions of men and women enjoyed each other's company prior to the discovery of mouthwash?

The truth is most of us do not have bad breath. A normal, healthy individual of any age has a normal clean breath, which is not offensive. According to Dr. Ray Allen Young, D.D.S., Arcadia, California, who has been in active dental practice for forty-five years and has stood with his nose near a patient's mouth about ninety thousand times, only two or three out of a thousand really have offensive breath.[1] In real cases of bad breath, mouthwash has no effect. Dr. Young says that with very few exceptions, bad breath does *not* originate in the mouth.

---

[1] Young, R. A., D.D.S., "Bad Breath Doesn't Need Mouthwash", *Prevention,* January, 1969

WHAT CAUSES BAD BREATH

In relatively few cases, bad breath *can* originate in the mouth and throat, caused by a tooth decay or serious infection in the gums or throat. But these conditions are comparatively rare and mouthwash would be of limited use in correcting them. They need proper medical and dental attention.

In the overwhelming majority of cases, the real causes of bad breath are in the digestive and eliminative tract. The unpleasant odor is caused by an exceptionally large amount of waste matter expelled through the lungs.

In the process of digestion and assimilation, great amounts of waste matter are created. These orginate chiefly in the stomach and small and large intestines, but waste matter also comes from every cell of your body. Each cell has its own metabolic system; it receives food and throws off waste. Via the bloodstream, this waste is transported to the various eliminative organs to be expelled.

HOW ODOROUS AND TOXIC WASTES ARE ELIMINATED

As a result of digestive and metabolic processes your body is always filled with large quantities of waste matter. Many of these wastes are odorous and most are highly toxic. If your body could not expel these wastes rapidly, you would die of self-poisoning in a very short time. Under normal conditions there is no danger of this happening. Your body is equipped with an extensive eliminative system. There are four basic eliminative organs—bowels, kidneys, lungs, and skin.

Although most of the waste matter is eliminated through the bowels and kidneys, the lungs and the skin are also effective. About one-third of all body waste is eliminated through the skin. The skin has been called the "largest eliminative organ," or the "third kidney." Hundreds of thousands of tiny sweat glands permit metabolic toxins to be excreted from the system. Uric acid, a normal compound of urine, is present in perspiration.

The lungs, too, are effective eliminative organs. When you inhale, they pick up oxygen and carry it through the blood to the cells. On its return, blood picks up waste matter from the cells and carries it back to the lungs where it is discharged on exhalation. Normally, the exhaled air is not offensive because the amount of odorous particles is too small to make the odor noticeable. Under some conditions, the bowels and kidneys are unable to eliminate all accumulated waste. When the kidneys and bowels do not function satisfactorily, part of their job is taken up by the skin and the lungs. The concentration of waste matter in the exhaled air will increase and you will have "bad breath."

CONSTIPATION—THE COMMON CAUSE OF BAD BREATH

Internal sluggishness and constipation are at the root of many evils. In addition to various pathological conditions such as rheumatic disease, gout, headache, skin disease and so forth, constipation can have a devastating effect on your complexion, which may assume a muddy tone. But by far the most conspicuous symptom of constipation is bad breath.

In order to understand how constipation can cause bad breath we have to familiarize ourselves with the digestive and eliminative tract and see how it functions.

Contrary to the average layman's notion, food is not digested in the stomach alone. Your food goes through a gradual process of digestion that starts in your mouth and ends in the large intestine and colon. As you chew, enzymes secreted by the salivary are acting on your food. As food enters the stomach it is subjected to a powerful working-over by several gastric enzymes and digestive secretions. Food continues through the small intestine, where still more enzymes further break it down and change it into a form which can be assimilated into the bloodstream. In the large intestine, bacteria work over the residual food particles. These bacteria also help manufacture various beneficial vitamins.

Your intestine contains billions of bacteria. Some of these are called "friendly bacteria," like the *acidophilus*; some "unfriendly." The latter are *putrefactive* bacteria. For optimum health, balance between these bacteria, often referred to as intestinal flora, is imperative. In good health, the correct bacterial balance is usually maintained as a matter of course.

But when your diet is unbalanced, stressing too much animal protein and over-refined constipating foods, and bowel movements are irregular due to a sedentary life, the balance of the intestinal flora will be disturbed. Harmful, unfriendly bacteria will take over and the result will be gas and putrefaction. Toxins created by bacterial metabolism and putrefaction may remain in the intestines and, as a result of prolonged constipation, be absorbed by the bloodstream where they threaten to poison the entire organism. In self-defense, your lungs try to purify the blood as it passes through. Thus, toxic and odorous impurities from the intestines are excreted with exhaled air, if they cannot escape in the natural way. The result is bad breath. When intestinal sluggishness and constipation become chronic, your halitosis will be chronic too. It's easy to grasp that this kind of bad breath—and most cases of bad breath do come from the lungs—cannot be improved or washed away by mouthwash.

A simple test may be made to prove the truth of the above statement. Swallow a few sealed garlic tablets and in a few hours you will have garlic breath. The garlic never touched your mouth, but via stomach and bloodstream it reached the lungs, to be excreted with the exhaled air. If you are told (by a good friend) that you have bad breath, ask him to check when you exhale through the nose, keeping the mouth tightly closed. You will find that the bad breath persists even when it completely bypasses the mouth.

MORNING BREATH

According to Are Waerland, the morning hours between four a.m. and noon constitute a period of elimination. At that time of day "the bloodstream is carrying the greatest burden of impurities, residues, and products of metabolism."[2] During the night your digestive and assimilative organs are busy selecting, distributing, and storing up nutrients for the coming day—the eliminative functions are slowed down considerably during the night. In the morning your system has accumulated large amounts of impurities and your bloodstream is heavily charged with waste products which the lungs are trying to expel.

Again, a perfectly healthy person has a clean breath even in the morning, just as all healthy children always have clean breath. "Clean as a child's breath," is an old saying based on actual observation. But if you are sluggish and constipated, and if you also drink coffee and alcohol and smoke tobacco, your blood will be filled with odorous residues which find their way out in the morning with exhaled air.

HOW TO PREVENT AND ELIMINATE BAD BREATH

Since your mouth is almost always innocent, mouthwash is not the answer to bad breath. Bad breath comes from

[2] Waerland, Are, HEALTH IS YOUR BIRTHRIGHT, Humata Publishers, Bern, Switzerland

within, the result of sluggish elimination, disordered metabolism, overeating, overworked kidneys and overloaded intestines, excessive smoking and drinking and other factors, most of which are within your control. In order to prevent and eliminate halitosis you must see that your general health condition is good and that your eliminative system is not overloaded or paralyzed by constipation. Here is a five-point program which can help solve your bad breath problem:

1. Avoid smoking and drinking.
2. Do not overeat. Overeating causes sluggish digestion, putrefaction in the bowels and accumulation of wastes in the system with a resultant bad breath.
3. Check with your doctor and dentist and make sure that there are no diseased conditions in your mouth, throat or respiratory tract.
4. Brush your teeth before going to bed with a soft brush and without toothpaste—just brush and rinse with plain water. Virtually all commercial toothpastes are harmful to the health of your teeth and gums. The regular use of mouthwash can be harmful to the delicate mucous membranes of your mouth.
5. See that your eliminative system works efficiently. If you are not having at least one bowel movement each day, you are constipated, whether or not you feel any immediate discomfort.

You can solve your constipation problem by observing the following simple natural rules of good elimination:

- Eat plenty of raw fruits and vegetables. Chew all your foods well.
- Avoid constipating refined carbohydrate foods, such as white sugar, white bread and baked goods.
- Eat six to ten soaked prunes with your breakfast. Be sure to drink the water in which the prunes were soaked.
- Supplement your diet with brewer's yeast, whey

powder, honey and yogurt—all natural laxatives.

- Exercise! Lack of exercise is one of the main causes of constipation. Plain walking is the best and easiest form of exercise.
- Consume plenty of liquids: water, juice (unsweetened only) soup.
- Never supress "nature's call." Try to establish at least two bowel movements a day, one upon arising and one before retiring. Be careful not to overstrain —relax and wait, if needed ten to fifteen minutes. This will eventually result in a well-established routine.
- Do not use commercial laxatives. They will only result in a degenerated and subsequently atrophied natural peristaltic rhythm.

If you follow the above program you will eventually achieve a normal and natural bowel rhythm.

A healthy person simply does not have bad breath. Therefore, make sure that your health is good and that your digestive and eliminative systems work efficiently. Then you can be reasonably sure, even without mouthwash or breathmint, that "if he kissed you once, he will kiss you again."

KEY POINTS IN THIS CHAPTER

1. The enjoyment of sexual union depends on both major and minor factors. Often, seemingly insignificant things such as smelly feet or bad breath can have a disastrous effect on amatory desire.

2. Contrary to some claims, bad breath only rarely originates in the mouth and thus cannot be improved by mouthwash.

3. Except in relatively few cases, bad breath originates in the digestive and eliminative tract, and offensive

breath odor comes from the lungs, which are trying to help the bowels and kidneys in their eliminative work.

4. The most common cause of bad breath is sluggish digestion and elimination; and consequent constipation.

5. A healthy person does not have bad breath. Bad breath is a symptom of faulty dietary patterns, ineffective digestion and putrefaction in the large intestine. These diseased conditions must be corrected before bad breath can be successfully and permanently eliminated.

6. Follow the five-point program outlined in this chapter and your breath will become clean and sweet—without mouthwashes, the prolonged use of which can be harmful for the delicate tissues of your mouth.

CHAPTER 16

ARE SYNTHETIC HORMONES IN FOOD TURNING AMERICAN MEN INTO EUNUCHS?

ACCORDING TO RECENT calculations, ninety per cent of our meat cattle and poultry are fed chemicals, drugs and/or synthetic hormones with their rations. These additives speed the growth and fattening time of the animals. Some seventy-five per cent of our cattle are fed or implanted with stilbestrol, a synthetic female hormone. About half the chickens and three-fourths of all beef on the market today have had stilbestrol treatments to speed their growth[1]—even though stilbestrol is known to have serious health-damaging potential. If you eat enough poultry and meat, you can be reasonably sure you receive a heavy dose of stilbestrol daily.

This synthetic female hormone has a disastrous effect on fertility and sexual libido in men. Even tiny amounts of this powerful drug have caused men to develop female characteristics. These hormones in meat have an effect on girls too, making them mature sexually before they normally

[1] Rodale, J. I., and staff, OUR POISONED EARTH AND SKY, Rodale Books, Inc., Emmaus, Penna., 1964

would be. A Bristish doctor, Leila Watson, said in *The Medical Officer* that the age of sexual maturity in girls has dropped from an average of seventeen to thirteen and a half. She suggested that hormone traces in chemically fattened meat are responsible.

Hormones are not the only factor draining our men of potency. The stresses of today's business and social rat race leave little energy for amatory interests. At the same time, our women, partly because of the widespread use of "the pill," are becoming more passionate and sexually oriented. This difference in sexual interest is ruining many marriages. Are we becoming the creatures that modern chemistry makes us? If so, chemistry is not doing as good a job as the original.

Many men look upon thick steaks as a source of strength and virility. This may—or may not—have been true once upon a time. Now the meat you eat contains sizable residues of drugs, hormones and antibiotics. Today's meat, stilbestrol-loaded, may be a cause of man's wilting potency.

HOW ITALIAN PLAYBOYS LOST THEIR MASCULINITY

Dr. George Belham relates an interesting example of what may happen when potent synthetic hormones are used indiscriminately. At a famous Italian seaside resort, the local beach playboys were known for their virility. A few years ago strange things began to happen. The local men, as well as male visitors who stayed at the resort for an extended period of time, found that their masculinity was rapidly disappearing. They became impotent and slightly effeminate. Their beards stopped growing. Even their breasts became enlarged and tender. Finally doctors were called to investigate this mysterious change.

The cause might never have been found had not one of the doctors, by sheer chance, found a tiny pellet in the breast of chicken on his plate. Chemical analysis showed that the pellet was a small stilbestrol (estrogen) pill.

A local poultry man had built a flourishing business with the help of hormone pellets and had succeeded in monopolizing production for the whole town, where grilled chicken was a popular dish in all restaurants, hotels and beach stands. He had implanted pellets in every bird soon after hatching, which helped to raise and fatten them in record time. Some part of the slowly dissolving pellet was still intact at the time of slaughter; and tourists as well as townspeople were consuming the pill with every portion of chicken. While the effect of this female sex hormone on the female population may have been to make them sexier, the effect on the males was disastrous.[2]

WHAT IS STILBESTROL AND HOW DOES IT CAUSE SEXUAL DISORDERS

Diethylstilbestrol is a synthetic hormone manufactured by chemical process. It has the properties of *estrogen,* a natural female sex hormone produced by the female sex glands. Estrogen plays a decisive role in the life cycle of a woman, including her normal sexual maturity. The master gland of the body, the pituitary, carefully regulates the amount of sex hormone produced and released. Too much or too little estrogen will cause havoc.

Stilbestrol fattens chickens and cattle just as castration does, and for the same reason. The drug will change a rooster into a capon. The comb and the wattle shrink; the bird becomes tame and lazy, the sex organs and glands dwindle and their activity declines. As a result of this alteration in sexual functions, the bird puts on weight rapidly. Stilbestrol forces the bird to achieve the size of an eight-month

---

[2] Belham, George, THE VIRILITY DIET, Dell Publishing Co., Inc., New York, 1968 Copyright (c) 1965 by George Belham

capon in five months. No wonder poultry men are happy with this discovery. As an executive for one of the largest feed manufacturers stated, "Stilbestrol is probably the most important happening in the cattle business in the past hundred years." In all this excitement over quick profits, the consumer who eats this medicated meat is left out of the picture. What happens to him, no one seems to care.

Once the most common way of using stilbestrol was to implant hormone pellets in the necks of chicken or the ears of cattle. In 1959 the government prohibited the use of implants in poultry, but farmers were still permitted to use stilbestrol implants on cattle and in poultry feed. The Canadian government, recognizing the serious danger of stilbestrol to health, prohibited the use of estrogen in any form for poultry or animals raised for food.

OTHER CHEMICALS IN MEAT

Stilbestrol is not the only harmful substance in meat. A goodly dose of antibiotics is added to feed quite regularly. The most frequently used are aureomycin and terramycin. Several arsenic-containing additives are also used in animal feed. Both antibiotics and arsenic compounds will improve the weight and speed the growth of the animals. Arsenic is, of course, a potent poison. The law requires that feed containing arsenic is not to be fed to animals five days prior to butchering. No controls exist to make farmers follow these regulations.

The animals receive various other drugs, including tranquilizers. Add to these the residues of toxic insecticides, such as DDT which is used on animals and in barns and chicken pens, and preservatives and synthetic flavorings and colorings, used in processed meats, and you will realize that the meat of today is not as it was twenty years ago—it is an adulterated food, loaded with a long list of toxic and harmful chemicals and drugs.

CHAPTER 17

CAN SMOKING CAUSE IMPOTENCE?

NOT ENOUGH DIRECT clinical research exists for a conclusive answer to the above question. Many well-known authorities on sex, however, have expressed the opinion that tobacco smoking has an adverse effect on the sexual urge and may be a cause of reduced potency. What research is available would tend to bear this out.

Dr. Magnus Hirschfeld believes that the potency of many smoking men is adversely affected by their habit.[1] He says that in some cases potency is restored when men cease to smoke. He explains that toxic substances in tobacco have a disturbing effect on the sex-hormone-producing chemistry of the body. Dr. D.W. Hastings, a well-known authority on impotency, reports that when some of his patients stopped smoking, they observed in themselves a markedly increased sexual drive.[2] Although not totally impotent before, they noted increased potency in a few weeks. Dr. Nor-

[1] As quoted in L. P. Wershub's SEXUAL IMPOTENCE IN MALE, Charles C. Thomas, Springfield, 1959

[2] Hastings, D. W., IMPOTENCE AND FRIGIDITY, Little, Brown & Co., New York, 1963

man Haire in THE ENCYCLOPEDIA OF SEX PRACTICE informs us that in some cases male potency was restored only after the patient stopped smoking.[3] A Russian researcher, Dr. Ilja Porudorninskij, reports that nicotine damages the sexual glands and the sexual nerve centers, and that excessive smokers can become impotent as a direct result of smoking.[4]

While many men smoke moderately and appear to have no problems as far as potency is concerned, many authorities believe that most heavy smokers suffer from some degree of weakened potency. The best way to find out what effect smoking has on your potency is to stop smoking for a few months and watch for a difference in the intensity and quality of your sexual drive.

Doctors from the University of Washington Medical School made a surprising discovery. Their research showed that women who smoke heavily are less likely to have male children than women who do not smoke. This statistic may be of only passing interest—but far more important and serious is the effect of smoking on the general health of the smoker.

The proper functioning of the genital apparatus in men as well as women depends on the condition of the entire organism which we call the human body. A sick man is generally disinterested in sex. Physical sickness of any kind is not conducive to amatory prowess. And there is no question that smoking is a definite cause of sickness.

It has been established that smoking can cause cancer, heart disease, emphyzema, stomach disorders and nervous conditions. Cancer and heart disease are major killers. Smoking is causatively involved in both.

---

[3] Haire, Norman, ENCYCLOPAEDIA OF SEX PRACTICE, Encyclopaedic Press Ltd., London, 1962

[4] "Excessive Smokers Can Become Impotent", *Tidskrift för Hälsa*, Stockholm, October, 1967

One of the worst effects of smoking is that it destroys vitamin C in your body. W.J. McCormick, M.D., the well-known authority on vitamin C, says that each cigarette destroys about twenty-five milligrams—the equivalent of the vitamin C content of one orange. This observation has been confirmed by research in Poland and the United States. Dr. McCormick says that in hundreds of actual tests of the vitamin C status of smokers, "a normal level of this vitamin has yet to be found."

What does this vitamin C destruction mean to your health? Vitamin C has a far-reaching effect. It will speed recovery from virtually any disease—from a simple cold to serious operations. Many researchers believe that vitamin C deficiency may cause a great number of our most common ailments, including arthritis and heart disease. Deficiency of vitamin C results in breakdown of the intercellular cement substance—collagen—and causes instability and fragility of the tissues. This may lead to a great variety of pathological developments.

Both the direct and indirect effects of tobacco smoking on health and sexual life—and particularly on man's potency—are too serious to be ignored or overlooked.

CHAPTER 18

WHAT ABOUT ALCOHOL AND SEX?

IN THE SEARCH through the ages for means and ways to improve his virility and stimulate his sexual interests, man has tried countless drugs, foods, herbs and drinks. High on the list of drugs considered effective in this respect is alcohol.

What is the truth about alcohol and sex? Does it have a stimulating effect on sexual desires or not? Does it improve sexual performance or does it have an opposite effect?

Basically alcohol is a sedative which inhibits and dampens physical and mental reactions. It has a twofold effect. In very small amounts it stimulates. Alcohol is a pure carbohydrate and is absorbed quickly into the bloodstream. It induces a feeling of well being by raising the blood sugar level. It also has a sedative, anesthetic effect by its paralyzing and inhibiting action on brain and nerve activity.

In numerous ancient writings, as well as in modern reports by such renowned authorities as Dutch gynecologist Th.H. Van de Velde, George Belham, Kenneth Walker and others, a certain degree of aphrodisiac property is attributed to alcohol in *small amounts*. Natural wines in particular are recommended for this purpose. Kenneth Walker advises a temporary use of small amounts of alcohol in cases of non-organic, or psychic, impotence to build up confidence. When, after a few successful performances, confidence has been restored, the use of alcohol should be discontinued.[1] It should be emphasized, however, that alcohol obviously has no aphrodisiac effect in cases of organic disorder.

It has been claimed that alcohol has also a favorable effect in cases of premature ejaculation. This may be because alcohol promotes muscular relaxation, reduces tension and also dulls the nerve responses.

ALCOHOL AND MALE POTENCY

But any beneficial effects of alcohol in relation to sex are greatly outnumbered by its harmful effects. A continuous use of alcohol, even in small amounts, will eventually bring about a gradual diminution of sexual capacity. In larger amounts alcohol definitely exerts a paralyzing action on the genital centers. Van de Velde states that *regular overindulgence* in alcohol leads to "extremely deleterious" effects on the genital organs and inhibits their normal functions.[2]

The adverse effect of alcohol on sexual potency has been affirmed recently by Dr. Alexander P. Runciman, researcher at the Reproductive Biology Research Foundation, St. Louis, one of the leading world centers for the scientific study of sex. Dr. Runciman, in his report to the recent clinical convention of the American Medical Association, said that excessive alcohol drinking can be blamed more than any other single factor for sexual impotence in males over fifty.

---

[1] Walker, Kenneth and Strauss, Eric B., SEXUAL DISORDERS IN THE MALE, Cassell and Co., London, 1954

[2] Van De Velde, Th.H., IDEAL MARRIAGE. Random House, N. Y., 1957

ALCOHOL—HEALTH DESTROYER

In addition to having a direct deleterious effect on the genital organs and their functions, alcohol has an indirect, long-range, harmful effect on sexual capacity by undermining the health of the individual. Alcohol causes premature aging by destroying one of the foremost "age-fighting" vitamins in the system—thiamine, or vitamin B_1. It has been clinically demonstrated that vitamin B_1 is closely linked with the aging processes of the body. Indispensable for the health of the nerves and brain, it is also an anti-fatigue vitamin. The French call it *joie de vie*—the-joy-of-life vitamin. Thiamine protects against stress and strain. Vitamin B_1 deficiency leads to fatigue and depression. Vitamin B_1 stimulates the sexual glands indirectly through its action on the pituitary gland.

Vitamin B_1 is used in the body in hundreds of different ways. One of its most important functions is to aid in the metabolism of carbohydrates. Pure refined carbohydrates, such as white sugar and white flour, cannot be effectively digested and used by the body without a sufficient supply of thiamine. All natural foods that contain large amounts of carbohydrates, also contain an ample amount of thiamine. Refined carbohydrates, such as white sugar and white flour, are totally lacking in vitamin B_1. For their proper digestion, the body must use its own stored B-vitamins. The body's storage is limited, however, and cannot last forever. A vitamin B-deficiency will soon result, with serious consequences.

Alcohol is a pure carbohydrate, totally void of B vitamins. Alcohol is made from fruits and grains which originally contained the important vitamins, but they were lost in the distilling and refining process. Alcohol will rob the body's own storage of vitamin B_1 and the continuous use of alcohol will result in a serious deficiency. It has been established that most organic diseases caused by alcohol are actually caused indirectly by thiamine deficiency.[3]

BEER AND WINE

A traditional belief exists that beer has a stimulating effect on sexual potency and can aid in the prolongation of coitus. No doubt the alcoholic content of beer and its ability to dull the nerves are responsible for this reputation. The common belief that beer is a "wholesome" drink no longer holds true—even if it was true in the past. Modern chemicalized beer has little resemblance to old-fashioned beer made of pure grains and containing valuable vitamins.

As to wines, a small glass of natural, mild, pure wine with a meal would, perhaps, not do much harm, and even might set the proper mood for a romantic evening. But natural pure wines are rapidly disappearing, especially in the United States. Most wines are fortified with pure spirits of alcohol, which is harmful in any amount.

ALCOHOLISM AND SEX

While moderate occasional use of alcohol may not cause serious harm, excessive habitual drinking will gradually destroy man's potency. Although alcohol in small amounts may seem a stimulant, the sexual escapades of drunkards are never of long duration. As a rule, a drunken individual is a poor lover. He is inconsiderate, his judgment is impaired and his potency seldom matches his appetite. But what is worse, alcohol acts as a poison on the genital tissues and organs and can bring about sterility and total atrophy of the reproductive system. Many scientists believe

[3] McCormick, W. J., M.D., *Archives of Pediatrics,* October, 1954

that even before alcohol can cause visible pathological changes and affect the health of the still young and healthy-looking drunkards, they find that their potency is all but gone.[4] Dr. Van de Velde writes that alcohol destroys the normal functions of testicles and causes insufficient production of spermatozoa.[2] Thus, an alcoholic gradually finds himself in an incurable situation of having lost both potency and fertility.

NUTRITION, ALCOHOL, AND SEX

If you drink and can't or don't feel that you should stop for social or other reasons, you can protect yourself from the harmful effects of alcohol by a few nutritional means. Alcohol robs your body of B-vitamins. Here's what you can do:

- Enrich your diet with brewer's yeast, the richest natural source of B-vitamins. Or buy B-vitamin tablets made from yeast and take as suggested on the bottle.
- Whole-grain products, wheat germ and liver are other excellent sources of B-vitamin complex.
- Avoid refined carbohydrates in the form of white sugar and white flour, and all foods made with them. Refined carbohydrates destroy B-vitamins in your system, just as alcohol does.

---

[4] Willy, A., M.D., et al., THE ILLUSTRATED ENCYCLOPEDIA OF SEX, Cadillac Publishing Co., Inc., New York, 1965

CHAPTER 19

CAN INSECTICIDES CAUSE STERILITY IN PEOPLE?

A FEW YEARS ago SILENT SPRING, the best-seller by Rachel Carson, shocked and alerted the nation to the harmful effects of poisonous insecticides on our health. The book deals primarily with the disastrous effect of poisonous chemicals on wild life—birds, fish and beneficial insects, like bees. In a few decades our poisons have succeeded in wiping out many entire species of birds, fish and insects. The American symbol, the bald eagle, has all but disappeared, while other strains are on the brink of extinction.

How do these chemicals work such disaster? Not as much, scientists agree, by direct toxic effect—although insecticides are extremely toxic—as by diminishing or destroying the fertility of the creatures that consume them.

What about the reproductive ability of human beings? Are we naive enough to believe that DDT and other potent poisons have a selective ability to affect the sterility of animals and birds, but not ourselves?

The American fertility rate has been going down for some years. In the last ten years, although a steadily increasing number of marriages was registered, our birth rate has dropped. At the same time, we are witnessing a continuous increase each year in the use of fertility-destroying chemicals in our food and environment. Some doctors estimate that twenty per cent of our men are already sterile and only forty per cent are highly fertile.[1] Recently, at the Annual Meeting of the American Chemical Society, Dr. R. M. Welch, of Tuckahoe, New York, voiced serious concern over the widespread use of pesticides and their effect on humans.[1]

HOW INSECTICIDES AFFECT FERTILITY

Animal experiments demonstrate that pesticides, even in small quantities, have a detrimental effect on the liver's enzyme-producing activity. Specifically, pesticides reduce the liver's production of the enzyme *dehydrogenase*. Dr. R. M. Welch has shown that the enzyme-inhibiting property in insecticides can also affect fertility. One of the functions of liver enzymes is to protect the sex hormones, testosterone and progesterone, from destruction in the general metabolic processes. When these enzymes are decreased, the sex hormones are destroyed. Continuous hormonal deficiency may result in infertility.

Dr. Welch, in extensive studies with male and female rats, demonstrated that insecticides in the diet cause sex hormone destruction. Three days after he added chlordane and aldrin to the diet of male rats, the seminal vesicles showed considerably lower than normal amount of testosterone, the male sex hormone. In similar experiments with female rats, Dr. Welch found that DDT, heptachlordane, and dieldrin—all frequently used pesticides—resulted in a reduced output of the female sex hormone, estrogen. He explains

[1] Farris, Edmond J., M.D., *Prevention,* January 1969

the harmful effect of insecticides by their ability to stimulate the estrogen destruction in the system.

These male and female sex hormones are vitally important not only for fertility, but also for general physical and mental development of the individual. They are responsible for the normal growth of sex organs and the maintenance of secondary sex characteristics. Deficiency may result in underdeveloped reproductive systems and in infertility.

Even very small amounts of pesticide—as little as one part per million—have a hormone-destructive effect.

Today our diets are loaded with insecticides. Dangerous residue levels have been found in milk, butter, meat products, vegetables and fruit. A recent test of restaurant foods in California showed that every food on the menu had traces of DDT. If pesticides can cut down the sex hormone levels in animals, why not in humans?

CHAPTER 20

WHAT CAUSES MALFORMED BABIES?

THE NUMBER OF miscarriages, stillbirths and malformed infants has been increasing during the past decade. Presently, seven per cent of children born alive in this country have some kind of abnormality. According to Dr. H. Nishimura, M.D., almost half of the population has some defect, if minor irregularities are included. Of the stillborn, ten to twenty per cent are malformed and forty per cent of early embryo deaths are associated with severe abnormalities.[1]

Are these abnormalities and malformations the "acts of God," as it once was common to think, or are they results of our modern civilized way of life? What role do our devitalized nutrition, rapidly increasing use of drugs and toxic food additives play? Can nutritional deficiencies cause miscarriages and the birth of defective or mentally retarded babies?

Dr. H. Curtis Wood, Jr., M.D., believes that certain abnormal conditions in newborn babies are not "acts of God," but are the result of a dietary lack in the pregnant

[1] Nishimura, Hideo, M.D., CHEMISTRY AND PREVENTION OF CONGENITAL ANOMALIES, Charles C. Thomas, Publisher, 1964

mother.[2] According to Dr. Wood, women in good nutritional status are better protected than others from the potential danger of miscarriage, premature labor, toxemia, labor abnormalities and abnormal conditions in the offspring. He cites vitamin C deficiency as a cause of pregnancy complications and a possible cause of certain congenital defects. As shown in hundreds of tests, pregnant women are likely to be low in vitamin C. This is especially true of women who smoke, because smoking destroys huge amounts of vitamin C in the body.

Recent tests made at the Pediatrics Clinic at the University of Tubingen, Germany, show that vitamin C is essential to milk-fed premature babies. A deficiency of vitamin C causes imbalance in amino acid metabolism, which can cause brain damage. A vitamin C deficiency in the mother may cause fragile blood vessels in the baby. Both the fetus and the nursed baby are dependant on the mother for their supply of vitamins and nutrients. To protect herself against the possibility of pregnancy complications and to prevent defects in her baby, the prospective mother should fortify her diet with large amounts of vitamin C.

Another factor in birth deformities is the growing use of dangerous drugs and x-rays. The thalidomide tragedy brought everyone's attention to the danger of potent modern drugs. But thalidomide is not the only drug that can cause birth defects. Some scientists believe that many more common drugs are involved in teratogenicity—the birth of deformed children. In England, some mothers who took *preludine*—an appetite-suppressing drug—gave birth to deformed babies.[3] The Canadian professor of genetics at McGill University, Dr. F. Clark Fraser, stated that hundreds of agents in our modern environment are harmful to the

---

[2] Wood, H. Curtis, Jr., M.D., OVERFED BUT UNDERNOURISHED, Exposition Press, Inc., N.Y., 1959

[3] *British Medical Journal,* November, 1962

mother and can damage the embryo. In addition to radiation and a variety of drugs (even some of the salicylates) Dr. Fraser pointed to dietary deficiencies, especially of vitamins B_2, A, E and folic acid, as possible causes of deformities in the newborn.[4]

B-complex vitamins are also essential. Research by Professor Bruno Filippi, of the University of Turin, and Dr. Charles Loux, of the University of Paris, two of the world's top experts in embryology, shows that vitamin B-complex deficiency can cause birth deformities. Further, a plentiful supply of B-complex not only helps prevent malformations but also protects the unborn baby against the teratogenic effects of drugs. Animal tests showed that malformations of the fetus, due to drugs such as antibiotics, do not occur if the supply of B-complex is adequate. Dr. Loux's research has demonstrated that a combination of riboflavin and pantothenic acid will protect the embryo against drugs. This suggests that an expectant mother, especially if she takes any kind of drugs, including prescribed medication, should include in her diet all the B-complex vitamins—particularly riboflavin and pantothenic acid.

Another nutritive factor in the reproductive process is vitamin E. In experiments reported by Dr. Bernard Baird of the University of California,[5] a definite relationship was demonstrated between oxygen supply during pregnancy and heart defects of newborn babies. It is well-known that vitamin E helps to oxygenate the blood and tissues. The fetus is in need of a constant oxygen supply. Smoking constricts blood vessels and hinders the flow of oxygen. An expectant mother should not smoke and, in addition, she should fortify her diet with vitamins C, B, and E.

A diet low in vitamin E can cause edema, skin sores and

---

[4] From the speech at the *Seminar on Birth Defects,* Ann Arbor, Michigan, 1962

[5] *Science News Letter,* June 13, 1964

blood changes in premature babies. These abnormalities improved when vitamin E was added to their formulas.[6] In other vitamin research at Ohio State University, concentrated wheat germ oil, rich in vitamin E, was given to 1,347 expectant mothers. Researchers reported that wheat germ oil reduced many of the complications of pregnancy as compared to the control group. The number of premature births was cut in half and the mothers on wheat germ oil delivered healthier babies. It should be noted that these favorable results were obtained from *wheat germ oil,* not the isolated vitamin E.

Even malformations caused by genetic defects may be forestalled by good nutrition. Unwanted hereditary traits are not invariably transmitted by parents, unless a so-called high degree of *penetrance* comes into play. Dr. Coda Martin, M.D, believes that good nutrition may prevent genetic defects by lowering the penetrance level[7] of abnormal genes.

All these studies show that poor nutrition in pregnancy will contribute heavily to congenital malformation and allied disorders. Diets deficient in many vital nutrients, plus the toxic environmental factors such as smoking, harmful drugs, and toxic elements in food, water and air are harmful to the mother and can damage the unborn baby. Dr. Fraser pointed out, at the seminar on birth defects, that diet deficiencies in themselves are enough to cause deformities in babies.

GOOD NUTRITION—A GUARD AGAINST BIRTH ABNORMALITIES

In summary, here is a nutritional program for preventing reproductive abnormalities.

---

[6] *John A. Hartford Foundation, Inc. Bulletin,* January, 1967

[7] Martin, Coda, M.D., A MATTER OF LIFE: BLUEPRINT FOR A HEALTHY FAMILY, The Devin-Adair Co., New York, 1964

1. "The use of *all* drugs during pregnancy should be restricted to the absolute minimum," says a German doctor, Professor Heinz Ruebsaamen of the University of Freiburg.

2. An expectant mother should have a diet rich in essential nutrients for her own and her baby's health. The basis of optimum nutrition diet is outlined in Chapter 9 of this book. The emphasis should be on *natural, unprocessed, unrefined* foods. Raw fruits, vegetables, whole grains, milk and milk products have the greatest potential for optimum health.

3. Smoking is incompatible with responsible motherhood. While I do not recommend anyone's smoking, an expectant mother should have the greatest motive for abstinence from tobacco.

4. Vitamin B-complex is essential for healthy pregnancy. A deficiency of B-vitamins in the mother's diet can cause congenital deformities in the baby. B-vitamins, especially riboflavin and pantothenic acid, shield the fetus from drugs which may cause birth defects. The best sources of B-complex vitamins are brewer's yeast, liver, wheat germ, milk, whole grains, nuts and seeds. Brewer's yeast and liver are the richest sources. Pregnant women should have one or two tablespoons of brewer's yeast each day as a protective dose.

5. The prospective mother's diet should be amply supplied with vitamin C. It will help to protect both mother and baby against the myriad of toxins in our food and environment. Fresh raw fruits and vegetables are best sources of vitamin C. Rose hips are the richest source; health food stores sell it. Plain ascorbic acid may also be used, but natural vitamin C in combination with the bioflavonoids, as it comes in rose hip tablets, is biologically more effective. The expectant mother should take 500 to a 1,000 milligrams of vitamin C throughout pregnancy—in case of threatened complication or problems, up to 1,500 and 2,000 milligrams a day would not be too much. Vitamin C is completely harmless and non-toxic.

6. Vitamin E is another vital factor in preventing reproductive disorders and birth defects. The best natural source of vitamin E is wheat germ oil. Expectant mothers should use one or two tablespoons of wheat germ oil daily. Wheat germ is also a good source of vitamin E, B-vitamins and proteins. In cases of threatened miscarriage, consult your doctor on the proper dosage of vitamin E in capsule form.

CHAPTER 21

HOW SAFE IS "THE PILL"?

MILLIONS OF WOMEN around the world are taking "the Pill" every day. It is estimated that 8½ million women use it in the United States alone. The oral contraceptive was developed some twelve years ago and its popularity has been steadily increasing. Most users take birth control pills without fear, convinced that they are harmless. One manufacturer distributes a brochure in which he states, "When taken as directed the Pill does not interfere with your state of well-being."

But how harmless is the Pill? Although most women—and many doctors—are unaware of it, evidence is mounting that oral contraceptives are potentially dangerous drugs which can play havoc with a woman's sexual and reproductive life and cause other serious disorders.

Here are a few things the Pill can do, according to reliable medical research:

- It increases the risk of death or disease due to blood clots by seven to ten times.
- It can cause liver damage and jaundice.

- It can cause "steroid diabetes" which can lead to clinical diabetes.
- It can cause sexual frigidity and loss of libido in some women.
- It can cause vaginal infections which can be transmitted to a man's penis during intercourse.
- It can cause visual disturbances, darker skin pigmentation and baldness.
- It may cause cancer in the breast.

THE PILL AND THROMBO-EMBOLIC DISEASE

Recent British studies reveal a seven to tenfold increase in death and injury due to thromboembolic diseases in women taking oral contraceptives.[1] The highest risk is for women between the ages of thirty-five and forty-four. There is higher incidence of *thrombophlebitis* (formation of blood clots and inflamation of blood vessels) and *pulmonary* embolism (the lodging of a blood clot in a vessel in the lung) among women who use oral contraceptives than among non-users.

Because of these studies, the FDA has requested that the Pill manufacturers state on the labels of birth control pills that they may be hazardous to health.

Almost from the start of its use, reports about circulatory complications caused by the Pill have come from various countries. Dr. J. H. Naysmith reported a death from coronary thrombosis of a thirty-three year-old British mother of six who was taking oral contraceptives.[2] A Bethesda, Maryland, mother with pulmonary embolism (clot in the lungs) swayed between life and death for three months after taking oral contraceptives. She was saved by anti-

[1] *New York Times,* May 11, 1968
[2] *The British Medical Journal,* January, 1965

coagulants.[3] After the shocking British report in early 1968, comparable studies were launched in the United States.

Recently, the British Medical Journal (March 1, 1969) reported that a safer oral contraceptive has been developed. Known in Britain as "the minipill" presumably it presents a lesser risk of blood clotting than the older, conventional types. The new Pill has been called "minipill" because it contains only one hormone—progesterone—instead of the usual estrogen-progesterone combination. Dr. Leon Poller, who reported the findings on minipill, warned however that further investigation will be needed to make sure the new pill is completely safe.

THE PILL AND LIVER DAMAGE

Reports have come from Finland, Sweden, Canada and the United States, indicating that oral contraceptives have been linked with jaundice in women users. Two Finnish doctors concluded their research by stating that the hormones in oral contraceptives are "the most important constituents causing liver damage."[4] Investigators in Santiago, Chile, reported a positive correlation between jaundice and oral contraceptives.[5] Many cases of clinical jaundice among women using the oral contraceptive *Anovlar* were reported from England.[6] Such reports, until recently, were usually dismissed both by the doctors and the patients who "believed in the Pill" as "unrelated coincidences."

Now, however, two American researchers from the Harvard Medical School, Dr. Robert K. Ockner and Dr.

[3] *Ladies' Home Journal,* July, 1967

[4] *The British Medical Journal,* October 31, 1964

[5] *The Lancet,* December 10, 1966

[6] *The British Medical Journal,* March 5, 1966

Charles S. Davidson, have conducted thorough studies and report a definite relationship between oral contraceptives and liver disorders.[7] Their microscopic studies of liver samples revealed that oral contraceptives, after being used for "two weeks to several months," can cause degeneration in the liver cells and jaundice. They describe the symptoms as the onset of malaise, anorexia, (loss of appetite), nausea, itching, dark urine and jaundice. They have demonstrated that cessation of contraceptive therapy usually resulted in the disappearance of symptoms within a few weeks to a few months. They reported that in two cases, when the contraceptives were readministered after remission, the jaundice recurred. Drs. Ockner and Davidson have ruled out the possibility of a simultaneously occuring liver disease or hepatitis. Their study demonstrated beyond reasonable doubt that the liver damage was caused by the ingredients in contraceptive pills.

THE PILL AND FRIGIDITY

Dr. William Masters is one of the world's leading sexologists. He is director of St. Louis' Reproductive Biology Research Foundation and the author of several books on sexual behavior and human sexual response. The first question Dr. Masters asks doctors and marriage counselors who refer patients to his clinic for frigidity is, "Has she been taking the Pill?" If the answer is yes, Dr. Masters insists that the patient stop using oral contraceptives for six months—in most instances the problem clears up during this time and no other measures are necessary.[8]

The other researcher who believes that prolonged use of

---

[7] *New England Journal of Medicine,* February 9, 1967

[8] *Insider's Newsletter for Women,* May 30, 1966

the Pill can cause secondary frigidity (failure to reach a satisfying climax) is Dr. J. E. Eichenlaub, a Minneapolis gynecologist. Dr. Eichenlaub told a Marriage Seminar in Kansas City, Missouri, that about twenty per cent of women feel a stronger sexual interest toward the end of their menstrual period, when there is a lower progesterone circulation in the system. When progesterone circulation is at its height, as during pregnancy or the beginning of the menstual period, they show a virtually complete disinterest in sex. The Pill spreads progesterone action through the system during the entire month and plays havoc with a woman's sexual responsiveness.[8]

OTHER ADVERSE SIDE-EFFECTS

According to Dr. Victor Wynn, director of the metabolic unit at St. Mary's Hospital in London, fifteen per cent of patients taking an oral contraceptive develop *"steroid diabetes,"* which can lead to clinical diabetes.[9] Dr. Wynn reported the following other contraindications (conditions when the Pill should not be used): hypertension, edema, family history of strokes or peripheral vascular or coronary disease, obstetric history of large babies, multiple stillbirths, congenital abnormalities and gross weight gain in pregnancy.

Studies reported by three California physicians indicate that some women may become relatively infertile when discontinuing the pills after a prolonged period of use.[10]

A British report links the Pill with an unusual scalp disease in which patches of hair fall out. Several instances of this disease occurred in women who had just started tak-

---

[9] *Medical Tribune Report,* February 5, 1968

[10] *Journal of The American Medical Association,* February 28, 1966

ing oral contraceptives.[11] A study by Dr. Frank Walsh, of John Hopkins University, showed that a number of women had developed visual disturbances after taking oral contraceptives.[12] Some of the Pill manufacturers include in their labeling a warning that the drug is contraindicated for patients with a history of stroke, bulging of the eye, partial or complete loss of vision and defects in the visual field or double vision.

Canadian studies showed a side effect from female oral contraceptives, which can affect men. An irritation and soreness of the penis was experienced by several men after sexual intercourse with women using oral contraceptives. Some women who use the Pill, it has been shown, suffer a vaginal infection and itch, vulvovaginitis, which can be transmitted to men.[13]

Two medical scientists, Dr. Robert W. Kistner, of Harvard Medical School and Dr. Saul Gusberg, chairman of obstetrics and gynecology of Mt. Sinai School of Medicine, warned recently that women taking birth control pills or the hormone estrogen (to prevent aging), risk development of breast cysts which may or may not lead to cancer. Estrogen has been used by women after menopause to prevent aging. Most oral contraceptives contain both estrogen and another female sex hormone, progesterone. Dr. Kistner said that one of the effects of estrogen is to produce an overgrowth of cells in the lining of the uterus. In a large percentage of women who develop cancer of the lining, the disease is preceeded by this overgrowth. Tests conducted in Chile have demonstrated that oral contraceptives can produce tumors in test animals who receive them regularly.[14]

---

[11] *The British Medical Journal,* October 23, 1965

[12] *Health Bulletin,* May 22, 1965

[13] *Canadian Medical Association Journal,* November 26, 1966

[14] *Nature,* December 12, 1966

THE PILL AND CANCER

In January 1970, several researchers warned U.S. Senate subcommittee that birth control pill may cause cancer. Dr. Marvin S. Legator, chief of the cell biology branch, U.S. Food and Drug Administration, said that because breast cancer lies dormant for many years it may be not detected for 10 or 20 years after the beginning of the pill use. Dr. Hugh J. Davis, the John Hopkins birth control specialist, said that the same synthethic hormones as used in the pill, have induced breast cancer in five different animal species. "Every important agent which has a carcinogenic (cancer-producing) effect in humans has been shown to cause cancer in animals. There is no reason to presume that the single exception to the transferability if such experiments will turn out to be the contraceptives," said Dr. Davis.

This short resume of research on the harmful side-effects of the Pill is not intended to create undue panic, but to emphasize that the Pill route to birth control is not as safe as many women think. While the majority of women seem to tolerate the Pill without noticeable discomfort, the risk nevertheless is very real for the minority who do not have that tolerance for one reason or another. In certain situations, the use of oral contraceptives appears to be warranted —for example, in the case of a mentally retarded young girl, or when pregnancy would present grave risks to health. But to make the Pill—this powerful and unpredictable hormone agent—a panacea for all birth control and population explosion problems, may turn out highly undersirable. The health risks connected with the Pill are too serious to ignore. It may be wise to exercise caution and use more cumbersome means of birth control and thus avoid the harmful side effects, the list of which continues to grow in medical literature.

CHAPTER 22

CAN AIR POLLUTION CAUSE REPRODUCTIVE DISORDERS AND DECLINE IN FERTILITY?

THE PUBLIC GROWS more and more aware of the danger of toxic insecticides in our food and environment. If insecticides can cause sterility in animals and birds, why not in people?

Also, much attention has been given recently to the ever-increasing problem of air pollution. Toxic substances in polluted air, notably carbon monoxide, have been pointed out as direct or contributing causes to many of our modern diseases—cancer, emphyzema and heart disease, to name a few. A California Institute of Technology biologist, Dr. A. J. Haagen-Smit, recently said that the oxide of nitrogen in our polluted air may affect the genes of generations to come. In his State of the Union address, January 22, 1970, President Richard Nixon called for a swift government action to clean our environment and preserve the health of this and the coming generations.

Although public awareness is growing in regard to toxic pesticides and industrial air pollutants, we hardly ever hear of one of the gravest of our environmental dangers—gradual but universal *lead-poisoning*. Many scientists are alarmed at the incredible speed with which lead is poisoning our environment.

Automobiles burn gasoline treated with lead, spraying the atmosphere with the substance. Lead then settles in the soil and on the crops, to be absorbed by fruits and vegetables. Crops that are grown near busy highways are particularly affected, since the air about them is filled with tiny particles of lead oxide. We are also constantly subjected to lead poisoning from industrial sources.

EFFECTS OF LEAD POISONING

Lead is one of the most toxic metals and even small amounts can be fatal. Because it is a cumulative poison, early symptoms are vague and hard to diagnose. In extreme cases, poisoning results in violent reaction and death. One child died after swallowing a lead button. The button dissolved rapidly in the system and caused fatal poisoning. But in most cases of gradual poisoning from polluted air and lead-poisoned foods, the symptoms are so well masked that they are often attributed to a virus or even emotional causes.

Symptoms may start with headache, loss of appetite and chronic fatigue. The person becomes nervous, irritable and tired. The system tries to eliminate poison through urine and feces, but if the system receives more than it is capable of eliminating, the poison is deposited in body tissues, especially the bones. Lead can adversely affect such organs as liver, kidneys, heart and nervous system.

As gradual poisoning continues, paralysis of the extremities may develop. Some doctors believe that the dreadful disease, multiple sclerosis, is caused by lead poisoning. Blindness, mental disturbance and even total insanity can be caused by lead poisoning.

Lead also has a detrimental effect on the reproductive

system. It interferes with fertility of both men and women and may cause miscarriage, premature labor, stillbirth and total sterility. Chronic lead poisoning can also cause sexual impotence.[1]

Again, acute lead poisoning is easy to identify, but chronic poisoning often remains undetected. It may require years of gradual poisoning for the effect to be unmistakable. Lead has a slow degenarative effect on the central nervous system and affects the genetic forces, as found by Russian scientists. A well-known toxicologist, Dr. Harriet L. Hardy, of the Massachusetts Institute of Technology, reported that mentally retarded children had higher levels of lead in the bloodstream than normal children.

WAS THE FALL OF ROME CAUSED BY LEAD POISONING?

According to American researcher, S.C. Gilfillan, Ph.D., there is no doubt that chronic, prolonged lead poisoning was the real cause of the Roman Empire's fall. Dr. Gilfillan tested the bones of the ancient Romans for lead content, studied their recipes and culinary customs, used modern methods of toxicology, archealogy and statistics to verify his conclusions. His findings suggest a gradual decline of fertility in the Roman aristocracy, due to the use of lead-lined utensils for food and wine. Lead also was widely used in water pipes, paint, cosmetics and toys.

How could this mass suicide go undetected? The Romans, apparently, never suspected that lead was poisonous. The poisonous property of copper was well-known. They avoided using it for food preparations, or lining utensils with it. Copper poisoning resulted in acute symptoms and the metal gave food an unpleasant taste. But the poisonous

---

[1]Willy, A., M.D., et al., THE ILLUSTRATED ENCYCLOPEDIA OF SEX, Cadillac Publishing Co., New York, 1965

property of lead was well hidden. The symptoms of lead poisoning were gradual, cumulative, and difficult to diagnose or identify.

Lead was used in astronomical amounts in Rome—over two million tons were produced in three hundred years. Water pipes and containers were made from lead. Food was cooked and served in lead utensils. Coins, toys, statuettes and buttons, were made of lead. Houses and furniture were colored with lead-containing paint. Roman wine contained large amounts of lead—and the Romans unknowingly added more lead to it in fourteen different ways.

Gradually, generation after generation, Roman health deteriorated, fertility declined and finally the greatest mass suicide in human history was an accomplished fact.[2]

HOW SERIOUS IS LEAD POISONING IN THE UNITED STATES?

Dr. Clair Patterson, geochemist of the California Institute of Technology, says that Americans are subjected to severe chronic lead poisoning and that the amount of lead in our foods and environment has reached the danger point.[3] It has been shown that vegetables from gardens in a small New York State town contain over one hundred parts per million of lead. This is thirty times more than the maximum permitted dose in canned goods. When tested, some pasture grasses near highways in Colorado contained seven hundred to three thousand parts per million of lead. The atmosphere in most parts of the United States today contains about a thousand times as much lead as pure air in the pre-smog era used to contain. It is estimated that in 1968 two hundred million pounds of lead entered the at-

---

[2] Gilfillan, S. C., Ph.D., *Technology and Culture,* 1961
[3] *Archives of Environmental Health,* September, 1965

mosphere from automobile exhaust pipes—or *one pound per capita!*

Dr. Wilfrid Bach, of the University of Cincinnati, said that if we continue to pollute air at the present rate, people will soon have to wear gas masks to survive!

Lead poisoning is not limited to the United States, of course. Most highly industrial countries face the same grave danger of systematic lead poisoning. In Germany, Switzerland, Russia and Sweden, scientists are alarmed at the speed with which the atmosphere, food and environment are becoming poisoned by lead. German scientist, professor Werner Schuphan, suggested that it should be forbidden by law to grow vegetables closer to the trafficked roads than five hundred meters (yards). In Sweden, several cases of lead poisoning were traced to vegetables from city lots. In the relatively quiet suburbs of Stockholm, curly kale grown in a backyard contained ten milligrams of lead per kilogram.[4] Swedish scientist Dr. W. Jenning considers this amount dangerous to health. Note that the vegetables grown in New York State contained eleven times that amount.

RUSSIA PROHIBITS LEAD IN GASOLINE

Most lead in our environment comes from the leaded gasoline used by automobiles. Russian scientists conducted an extensive study of environmental lead poisoning and, as a result, in 1956 the Russian government totally banned lead in gasolines. In the United States there is no such restriction. Lead is, of course, used to make high octane automotive fuel. High octane gasolines *could* be made without lead. Amoco, the American Oil Company's gasoline, is produced without it. But most fuel industries are more concerned with their profits than with the people's health.

---

[4] Svenson, Eskil, *Tidskrift för Hälsa,* Stockholm

HOW YOU CAN PROTECT YOURSELF FROM LEAD POISONING

Lead contamination of our foods and environment is almost universal. If you live in a city you are exposed to lead constantly, from automobile exhausts, from industrial plants, from lead in water and foods, from smoking of tobacco. It has been estimated that the average city-dwelling American absorbs about thirty micrograms of lead daily from food, drink and air. If you smoke, you have ten additional micrograms.[5]

Fortunately, you have a few ways of protecting yourself from lead poisoning.

First, extra supplies of calcium in your diet have both preventive and curative effect on lead poisoning. Lead is usually deposited in the bones. Some studies show that less lead is absorbed and more is safely excreted, when the system had a plentiful calcium supply before exposure. Also, some findings in England indicate that calcium and vitamin D injections help in recovery from acute lead poisoning. Calcium has a protective property against other toxic substances, for example, strontium 90. You would be wise, therefore, to fortify your diet with extra amounts of calcium and of vitamin D, which helps the body to assimilate calcium. Bonemeal tablets or powder are good sources of easily assimilable calcium. Cod liver oil is a good natural source of vitamin D.

Other substances found useful in protection against lead poisoning are vitamins C and thiamine (B_1).[6] Vitamin C is, of course, the anti-toxin vitamin. Rose hips, citrus fruits and other fresh fruits and vegetables are the best

---

[5] "Lead—the Inescapable Poison", *Prevention,* December, 1968

[6] *Tohoku Journal of Experimental Medicine,* 46; 295:322, 1944

natural sources of vitamin C. Vitamin C must be taken in large amounts as a protective dose against toxic effects of lead—1,000 mg. or more a day. To obtain this amount of vitamin C you must use it in tablet form.

It took eighteen generations of severe lead onslaught to wipe out the Roman aristocracy. We have reason to fear that the present lead onslaught is doing a more rapid and thorough job. The Romans were destroyed by their ignorance. If we are destroyed by lead poisoning, at least we can't blame our ignorance for it.

VITAL POINTS IN THIS CHAPTER

1. Widespread systematic lead poisoning is one of the gravest dangers to health in today's industrialized society.
2. Lead is a powerful, cumulative toxic agent, which can cause many health disorders, including sterility. Chronic lead poisoning can cause male impotence.
3. The fall of Rome was brought about by chronic, prolonged lead poisoning, which caused a gradual decline in fertility.
4. Americans are constantly subjected to severe lead poisoning, mainly because of the lead-treated gasolines burned by our automobiles.
5. The total ban of lead in gasolines and industry would prevent a repetition of the Roman tragedy. Meanwhile certain nutritional means can help you protect yourself against the universal danger.

CONCLUSION

Scientific inquiry has just started into the relationship between sex and nutrition. The veil of inhibitions and taboos has been lifted. Doctors are delving into the biological and nutritional aspects of sexuality with exploratory zeal. In several research centers in the United States as well as many other countries, dedicated men are seeking the answers to unanswered questions in this area. In years to come we will undoubtedly have solid facts in many areas where we now can only hypothesize.

In this book you have learned that your sexuality is closely tied to your general health; and that the condition of your health is inseparably tied to the quality of your nutrition. You have learned that a well-balanced diet of natural, unprocessed foods and certain food substances—vitamins, proteins, minerals, trace elements—can enhance your sexual vigor and improve your physical capacity for love. Conversely, devitalized nutrition, and other health-destroying environmental factors of modern life, present a grave threat to your health generally, as well as to your fertility and sexual vigor.

The purpose of this book is to help you understand yourself, your desires and urges, and to make you aware of the relationship between them and your mode of living. Nutrition is not a panacea, or cure-all. Furthermore, nutrition does not compete with medical practice. Your own effort to improve your health by better nutrition does not mean self-doctoring. By discarding poor living and eating habits, however, you demonstrate an intelligent and responsible attitude toward your health.

Building health through improved nutrition is not as easy as it may seem. Health knowledge is of no use unless it is put into practice, which involves understanding, determination and willingness to change your health-destroying habits. New eating habits and health-promoting ways of living must be strictly adhered to. Often, it may take time before noticeable results can be obtained. It may have taken decades of nutritional abuse to ruin your health and lower your vitality and virility; it may take months and years before health and vitality can be totally restored.

Naturally, I do not profess that improved nutrition will miraculously solve all the sexual problems of mankind. Deep-seated fears and inferiority complexes, based on unsuccessful experiences, misconceptions and inhibitions, can have a devastating effect on sexual life. Such psychological problems can be solved only by uncovering and eliminating the underlying causes.

On the other hand it has been demonstrated that improved nutrition can build a solid basis not only for better physical health but also for improved mental and emotional health. Optimal nutrition will re-activate glandular functions which, in turn, can have a most positive rejuvenating and revitalizing effect on man's whole personality, his emotional feelings and desires, his will and ability to face problems and his strength to solve them. I can imagine no sounder basis than physical and emotional health for happier marriage and greater sexual fulfillment.